Review of Surgery

Review of Surgery

Amit Goel

DA MS (Gen Surgery) FICS FNB (Minimal Access Surgery)

Assistant Professor
Department of Surgery
Army College of Medical Sciences
New Delhi

CBS

CBS Publishers & Distributors Pvt Ltd

New Delhi • Bengaluru • Chennai • Kochi • Kolkata • Mumbai
Bhubaneswar • Hyderabad • Jharkhand • Nagpur • Patna • Pune • Uttarakhand

Review of
Surgery

ISBN: 978-81-239-2200-3

First Edition: 2012

Reprint: 2018

Published by Satish Kumar Jain and Produced by Varun Jain for
CBS Publishers & Distributors Pvt Ltd
4819/XI Prahlad Street, 24 Ansari Road, Daryaganj, New Delhi 110 002, India.
Ph: 23289259, 23266861, 23266867 Website: www.cbspd.com
Fax: 011-23243014 e-mail: delhi@cbspd.com; cbspubs@airtelmail.in.

Corporate Office: 204 FIE, Industrial Area, Patparganj, Delhi 110 092
Ph: 4934 4934 Fax: 4934 4935 e-mail: publishing@cbspd.com; publicity@cbspd.com

Branches

- **Bengaluru:** Seema House 2975, 17th Cross, K.R. Road, Banasankari 2nd Stage, Bengaluru 560 070, Karnataka
  Ph: +91-80-26771678/79 Fax: +91-80-26771680 e-mail: bangalore@cbspd.com
- **Chennai:** No. 7, Subbaraya Street, Shenoy Nagar, Chennai 600 030, Tamil Nadu
  Ph: +91-44-26680620/26681266 Fax: +91-44-42032115 e-mail: chennai@cbspd.com
- **Kochi:** 42/1325, 1326, Power House Road, Opposite KSEB Power House, Ernakulam 682 018, Kochi, Kerala
  Ph: +91-484-4059061-62-64-65 Fax: +91-484-4059065 e-mail: kochi@cbspd.com
- **Kolkata:** No. 6/B, Ground Floor, Rameswar Shaw Road, Kolkata-700014 (West Bengal), India
  Ph: +91-33-2289-1126, 2289-1127, 2289-1128 e-mail: kolkata@cbspd.com
- **Mumbai:** 83-C, Dr E Moses Road, Worli, Mumbai-400018, Maharashtra
  Ph: +91-22-24902340/41 Fax: +91-22-24902342 e-mail: mumbai@cbspd.com

Representatives

- **Bhubaneswar** 0-9911037372 • **Hyderabad** 0-9885175004 • **Jharkhand** 0-9811541605 • **Nagpur** 0-9021734563
- **Patna** 0-9334159340 • **Pune** 0-9623451994 • **Uttarakhand** 0-9716462459

Printed at Goyal Offset Printers, GT Karnal Road, Industrial Area, Delhi, India

Preface

Review of Surgery has been written to facilitate students for a quick revision of surgery before their professional examinations. As teaching faculty at a medical college, I came across the difficulties of undergraduate medical students that inspired me to write this book. It covers the entire syllabus of surgery in the form of short notes, question-answers, and practical tips for the examinations. This book would help students of surgery in theory, practical and preparation for postgraduate medical entrance examinations. It gives me immense pleasure and happiness to present this book to medical students, the efforts for which started two years back. Before examinations, course is vast and time is short, and this book would help the students to revise the course in a short time.

I would like to thank CBS Publishers & Distributors and their staff who have made sincere efforts in the publication of this book.

Amit Goel

email: gamit11@rediffmail.com

to

my wife

Dr Ruchi Goel

and son

Saumaya Goel

Contents

1 Introduction and Anaesthesia

The practice of surgery demands a logical, methodical approach that requires a round knowledge of anatomy, physiology and pathology of any condition encountered. Understanding and presentation are the key to success in any examination.

The basis of all pathologic processes requires a clear definition of the condition.

Features of condition that need to be described

Incidence
Age
Sex
Geography
Aetiology
Pathology
Macroscopic/microscopic appearance
Management
Staging/spread
Prognosis

The mnemonic which outlines it "In a surgeon's crown, a physician might make some progress".

Management describes the process of diagnosis (history/examination), specific tests for investigation and treatment.

Describe the detailed history, examination and proposed investigation and presumptive differential diagnosis whenever student is asked to describe or present a case. Therapy should include treatment modalities, prevention and education.

General measures should include rest, hygiene, diet, pharmacological agents, nursing, support therapy and therapeutic modalities follow-up.

One should describe and classify conditions into:

- Infective
- Neoplastic
- Drugs
- Iatrogenic
- Collagenosis
- Autoimmune
- Traumatic
- Idiopathic

- Vascular
- Endocrine or environmental
- Psychological
- Metabolic

Infective procedures can be further divided into bacterial, viral, fungal, parasitic, spirochaetal rickettsial, retroviral. Complications should always be described in terms of general and specific complications.

HISTORY

It is much debated issue and should form a part and parcel of every procedure and has medicolegal implications. All complications should be clearly described to patient and recorded on the consent form.

Work up of Patient

1. Detailed history
   - Present and past history
   - Drug history
   - Allergies
   - Family history
   - Social history
   - Gynaecologic and obstetric history

For Example

Taking history of pain one can define as–Mnemonic Socrates

- **S**ite
- **C**haracter
- **A**ssociation
- **E**xacerbation
- **O**nset
- **R**adiation
- **T**iming
- **S**everity

2. Examination
   - General condition
   - Cardiovascular system
   - Abdomen
   - Mental and Physical State (CNS)
   - Chest
3. Investigations
   - Basic investigations like function tests. Haemogram, kidney function test that X-ray chest, ECG, serum electrolytes.
   - Specific investigations

   Preoperative preparation

   - After history, examination, tests marking the site, marking the side and specific preoperative preparation for specific surgery.
     Example: Bowel preparation for colonic surgery.

Antibiotics for prophylaxis is to be given placement of tubes like urinary catheter to decompress bladder, nasogastric tube.

Medical management of systemic conditions like diabetes, heart diseases, chronic obstructive pulmonary disease (COPD) should be routinely done.

Operative Steps

- It should include description of anaesthetic technique local or regional, position of patient, e.g. midline prone lithotomy, etc.
- Skin preparation should describe antisepsis, draping and toweling, position of surgeon and assistants and in case of laparoscopy, the position of camera and monitor as well operative steps should mention the approach entering tissue planes, findings of diagnostic laparotomy or laparoscopy, pathology or coexisting pathologies, detailed procedure. One should also describe detailed closure with details of haemostasis, drainage, suture material, swab and instrument check.

Example: Postoperative management should include fluid and electrolyte and nutrition management, administration of antibiotics or other drugs, timings for removal of draw sutures, dressings, investigation specific nursing instructions like detailed parameter and input/output and nutrition chart specimen for histology and microbiology, radiology reports and date and time of discharge and subsequent follow-up.

Example

Suture material	*Absorbable*	*Nonabsorbable*
Monofilament	1. Surgical gut • Plain • Chromic 2. Collagen • Plain • Chromic 3. Monocryl 4. PDS II 5. Polyglactin	1. Polyamide 2. Polypropylene 3. Stainless steel 4. Polyester
Multifilament	1. Polyglycolic acid 2. Polyglactin 910 3. Polyglactin 910 Rapid	1. Surgical silk 2. Surgical linen 3. Cotton 4. Polyamide 5. Polyester 6. Stainless steel

Synthetic absorbable sutures like vicryl rapid, monocryl, etc. Needles can be eyed or eyeless round bodies, uppercut and cutting or micropoint of special needles like tapercut needles.

WOUND HEALING AND INFECTION

Definition: The term **Healing** refers to the replacement of destroyed tissue by living tissue.

The healing process has two aspect:

A. ***Contraction:*** A mechanical reduction in the size of the defect occurring in the first few weeks.

B. ***Replacement of lost tissue:*** This is brought about by:

a. Migration of cells

b. Multiplication of adjacent cells to provide extra time to fill the gap. This is accomplished in two ways:

- *Regeneration:* Replacement of lost tissue by tissue similar in type due to the proliferation of surrounding undamaged specialized cells.
- *Repair:* The replacement of lost tissue by granulation tissue, which matures to form scar tissue. This is inevitable when the surrounding specialized cells do not posses the capacity to proliferate, e.g. muscles and neurons.

Wound healing is a complicated process involving:

- Movement of cells
- Division of cells
- Rearrangement of tissues
- Biochemical changes

In healing the phases are as follows:

1. *Lag phase:* For a few days no marked changes are seen in the wound.
2. *Rapid change in size due to contraction:* Biochemical changes take place in the early period. On Microscopic examination there is an acute inflammatory reaction, initially and rapid cell division is occurring later.

The basic that happen in wound healing are:

1. Wound contraction
2. Granulation tissue formation
3. Biochemical changes

1. Wound contraction

a. *Lag phase:* Initially for 2–3 days followed by

b. *Period of rapid contraction:* Which is largely completed by the 14th Day. The wound is reduced by approximately 30% of its original size. Contraction of the wound results in much faster healing as 1/4th to 1/3rd amount of new tissue have to be formed.

Causes of wound contraction: No definite causes are known, but the accepted ones are:

1. Removal of fluid by drying.
2. Contraction of collagen: It is supposed that the contraction mechanism lies in the edge of the wound. Interference with this area delays contraction.

Preoperative care

- Proper diagnosis
- Informed consent

- Preoperative evaluation of cardiorespiratory system, exercise tolerance, illness, drugs allergy
- Type of anaesthesia/analgesia
- Investigation

ASA (American Society of Anaesthesiologists)

1. Normally healthy
2. Mild systemic disease
3. Severe systemic disease
4. Incapacitating disease
5. Moribund

Preoperative preparation

- Fasting
- Bowel and skin preparation
- Investigation
- DVT prophylaxis Fragmin 5000 SC before surgery and compression garments.
- Prophylactic antibiotics

Anaesthesia

- Premedication
- Patients are administered general anaesthesia, regional anaesthesia
- Local anaesthesia is by giving lignocaine 3 mg/kg and 7 mg/kg if adrenaline is mixed, bupivacaine 2 mg/kg.

Postoperative Complications

Pyrexia: Lung collapse, infection, anastomotic leak, UTI blood culture cannulations meningism, endocarditis and deep vein thrombosis.

Pain: Narcotic analgesics like morphine nonsteroidal NSAIDs.

Hypoxia: Pneumonia, pulmonary embolism, lung collapse, pneumothorax, fasting blood culture, arterial blood gases, X-ray chest and ECG.

Hypotension: Oxygen, hypovolaemia to be managed cardiogenic causes like embolism, inspiration, anaphylaxis and sepsis.

Nausea/Vomiting: Ileus, emetic drugs like opiates, digoxin, nasogastric, anaesthetic drugs and antiemetics.

Oliguria: Output should be 50 ml/hr replacement of lost fluid, shock nephrotoxic drugs and transfusion trauma, and fluid retention.

Day care surgery: Do not discharge until **LEAPFROG** is established.

L Lucid, not vomiting, cough reflex
E Easy breathing, urination
A Ambulant
P Pain relief
F Follow-up, removal of drain
R Rhythm like pulse, BP

O Operation site checked
G GP orders

Approach to Examination

Initial impression: Appearance and mannerisms, speak clearly and loudly

The acronym **PLANT** can be used to answer

PAUSE

LISTEN

ANALYSE

NOTE

TALK

QUESTIONS AND ANSWERS

1. **What is suture?**

   Ans: Any strand of material used to ligate blood vessels or approximate tissues.
2. **What are types of sutures?**

   Ans: Absorbable and nonabsorbable.
3. **What are catgut sutures and two types of catgut sutures?**

   Ans: Purified collagen from intestines of cows and sheep, plain catgut and chromic catgut treated with chromium.
4. **What is suture?**

   Ans: Absorbable, braided, multifilamentous copolymer of lactide and glycoside.
   It retains strength 60% 2 weeks, 8% 4 weeks.
5. **What is PDS?**

   Ans: Absorbable monofilament of polydiaxanone. 150 days absorption period.
6. **What is silk?**

   Ans: Branded protein filament spleen by silkworm larva.
7. **What is prolene?**

   Ans: Nonabsorbable suture.
8. **What is vertical mattress and horizontal mattress?**

   Ans: Far-far, near-near vertical mattress and horizontal mattress sutures is taken, needle is reversed and same bite is taken again parallel to wound.

2

Shock

Shock is defined as a state in which the metabolic demands of the cells are not met by the supply of nutrition from the body leading to state of acute systemic hypotension in which there is:

a. Persistent deficiency of blood flow through the peripheral vascular system.
b. Decreased perfusion of vital organ.

It leads to pallor, weakness, sweating, rapid therapy, pulse, oliguria, cyanosis, restlessness, apprehension followed by confusion.

PATHOPHYSIOLOGY OF SHOCK

Shock leads to decrease in intravascular volume, low cardiac output, vasoconstriction, tachycardia, decreased renal flow.

Juxtaglomerular apparatus detects decreased blood pressure, stimulating release of renin which is converted to angiotensin causing peripheral vasoconstriction and stimuli release of aldosterone which leads to elevated peripheral vascular resistance which raises systolic blood pressure, increases intravascular volume and leads to sodium and water retention leads to increased secretion of anti-diuretic hormone, renal absorption of water. Metabolic acidosis due to tissue metabolism which is anaerobic leads to lactic acid production. Potassium retention present in patients with decreased renal function.

Major Causes of Shock

1. Anaphylactic
2. Cardiogenic
3. Hypovolaemic
4. Bacteriogenic
5. Neurogenic
6. Adrenal insufficiency

Treatment Goal

To restore adequate tissue perfusion and oxygenation oxygen delivery:

Measurement of cardiac output

- Oesophageal Doppler
- Lithium dilution
- Impedance cardiography

Condition	BP	Pulse cm^{-5}	PCWP mm Hg	CI m^2	SVR dym/sec	O_2D ml/nm	O_2L ml/nm
Normal (N)	120/80	80	5–15	2.5–3.5	1000–1500	900–1200	200–300
Hypovolemic	↓	↑	↓	↓	↑	↓	↓
CHF	↑	↑	↑	↓	↑	↓	↓
Cardiogenic shock	↓	↑	↑	↑↓	↑↓	↑↓	↑↓
Septic shock	↓	↑	↓ or N	↑	↓	↑	↑ or N
Neurogenic shock	↓	↑ or N	↑ or N	↓ or N	↓	↑ or N	N

BP arterial blood pressure, P pulse, PCWP pulmonary capillary wedge pressure, CI cardiac index, SVR systemic vascular resistance, O_2D oxygen delivery, O_2L oxygen consumption

HYPOVOLEMIC SHOCK

Most common form of shock due to loss of whole blood, plasma, electrolytes and water. It leads to reduction in oxygen delivery resulting from diminished cardiac output.

Phase I: Venous reservoirs normally containing 70% of total blood volume are depleted 500 ml that is lost is compensated.

Phase II: Fall in systemic arterial blood pressure when 500–1000 ml of blood is lost. Systemic BP may fall to 90 mm Hg blood pressure will return to normal within hours. If 1000–2000 ml are lost, the blood pressure falls and if it remains low for 24–28 hours, secondary effects like renal failure, cyanosis start.

Phase III: Volume loss greater than compensation, repeated continuous bleeding cardiac output reduced, may lead to acute respiratory failure of sudden relaxation of constructed venous reservoirs.

Treatment

1. Replacement of losses by fluid.
2. Patients who have lost blood need to have blood replacement along with crystalloids.
3. High molecular weight dextran or colloids can be used as substitute for plasma. lactated Ringer's, normal saline are good balanced electrolyte solutions.
4. If fluid resuscitation to be assessed by invasive central lines (CVP and Swan and Ganz), as well as urinary output, mental function, blood pressure and heart rate.
5. Correction of underlying problem whether an intra-abdominal process or injuries.
6. It is possible to replace 75% of whole blood loss by crystalloid solutions. Large enough quantities are given. 1 ml loss or red cell mass should be replaced by 1 ml of electrolyte solution; 1 ml of plasma lost should be replaced with 3 ml of electrolyte solutions. Thus when a man of 70 kg loses 4000 ml of blood, 12 litres of electrolyte solution are required.
7. If hypovolemia from whatever cause is not adequately corrected, it becomes refractory which causes physiology changes such as:
   - Pooling of blood in microcirculation
   - Adrenocortical insufficiency

- Shock lung
- Superimposed cardiogenic or septic shock.

CARDIOGENIC SHOCK

A. Causes

1. Massive myocardial infarction
2. Acute aortic/mitral regurgitation
3. Post cardiac surgery
4. Traumatic myocardial contusions
5. Pulmonary embolism.

B. Effects

1. Cold, clammy, skin sweating, tachycardia, hypotension
2. Pulmonary oedema
3. Cardiac arrhythmias and metabolic acidosis.

C. Management

Maximal myocardial performances with oxygen. It is dependent on degree of damage to myocardium. Treatment is mainly supportive like:

- Oxygen, ventilation
- Optimise PCWP (better guide than CVP, aim for 16–20 mm)
- Relief of pain
- Balloon pump (intra-aortic)
- Decrease after load with diuretics and vasodilators and increase contractility with dopamine.

SEPTIC SHOCK

Septic shock can be due to gram-positive organisms, gram-negative organisms, fungi, protozoa. Both sepsis and non-septic events (trauma, ischaemia, haemorrhage, pancreatitis) can induce systemic inflammatory response syndromes (SIRS).

1. Disseminated macrophage and neutrophil activation
2. Mediator release
3. Endothelial damage
4. SIRS can manifest by two or more of following
5. Temp >38°C
6. Heart rate >90/min.
7. Respiratory rate >20/min or PCO_2 <4.0 kPa
8. White blood count >12,000/min^3.

Pathology

Activation of complement system cytokines, arachidonic acid metabolites, platelet activating factors, histamine, nitric oxide can lead to vasodilatation, increased capillary permeability, poor cellular oxygen utilization and myocardial depression.

A. Early septic shock/hyperdynamic warm shock
   1. Most commonly manifested in positive organisms but rarely gram-negative and fungal array also be involved.
   2. Hypotension, tachycardia but patients are warm and pink.
   3. Increased cardiac output. Late septic subsequently C decreasing. Myocardium function, cardiac output decreases, profound fall in BP, fever, rigors and cyanosis.
   4. Vasoconstriction causes cool extremities.
   5. End result is cellular hypoxia and multiple organ dysfunction syndrome. This is cold septic shock.

Treatment

1. Treatment of endotoxic shock by general measures, e.g. draining of pus or removing infectious broad spectrum antibiotics therapy.
2. Treatment of underlying etiology, management of haemodynamic gets with adequate oxygenation and cardiovascular support with noradrenaline 0.01–0.2 mcg/kg/min and renal support like hemofiltration if required.

Monitoring of patients by pulse oximetry, cardiac status, urine output and arterial blood gas analysis.

Inotropic Drugs

Drug	*Dose mcg/kg/min*	*Receptor*	*Effects*
Dopamine	0–5	Dopaminergic	Renal/Mesenteric vasodilator: GFR 0–10 β_1 increased cardiac output, BP >10 α_1 IV vasoconstriction
Dobutamine	2.5–15	$\beta_1 > \beta_2$	Myocardial contractility. Reduced left ventricular and diastolic pressure and action is seen only when β is blocked.
Adrenaline	0.01–0.2	$\beta_{1+2} - \alpha$	Increased cardiac output β_1 vasodilatation β_2
Enoximone	Phosphodiesterase	Inhibitors	Increased myocardial contractility

NEUROGENIC SHOCK

1. Hypotension secondary to CNS dysfunction.
2. It is commonly seen in trauma, pneumothorax and cardiac tamponade.
3. Results from absorption of sympathetic nervous system due to widespread vasodilation.

Treatment

Involves place patients in Trendelenburg's position using intravascular volume replacement or giving sympathomimetic agents to improve peripheral vasoconstriction.

ANAPHYLACTIC SHOCK

1. Mainly due to reactions specially penicillin group of drugs.
2. Basic cause is liberation of histamine and widespread dilatation of capillaries together increase in capillary permeability cause blood to the pooled in microcirculation. There can be bronchospasm, rashes, hypotension. Treated by 0.5 ml to 1 ml of adrenaline IV of IM. Administer oxygen and fluids.

Fluid

Preoperative: Dehydrated patients should be resuscitated before anesthesia as it compounds shock.

Postoperative: Two to three liters of fluid requirement/24 hr and standard regime is 2 liters of 5% dextrose with 1 liter 0.9% saline.

Dehydration : Increase by 5 liters if severe
Shock : 0.9% saline fluid of choice
Loss from gut : Replace NG with 0.9% saline
Transpiration losses : Burns and fever

Low blood pressure is due to inadequate fluid infusion. Increase IV fluid and fluid challenge of ½-L liters.

Renal failure : Given 500 ml + previous day's output
Heart failure : Half the volume 1–5 liters/24 hr. Avoid sodium, use 5% dextrose
Hypovolemic shock : Crystalloid–do not stay as long in intravascular compartment
Colloid : They equilibrate with total extracellular volume.
Keep haematocrit of 0.3 and urine >30 ml/hr.

QUESTIONS AND ANSWERS

1. Cardiac output is increased by
(a) Endotaxemia and shock
(b) Hypervolaemia
(c) Pneumothorax
(d) Sympathetic stimulation
(e) Altitude

(a) T (b) F (c) F (d) T (e) T

2. Systemic circulation vasodilators include
(a) Calcium channel blockers
(b) Ischaemia
(c) Carbon dioxide
(d) Glyceryl trinitrate

(a) T (b) T (c) T (d) T

3. Pre-renal failure
(a) It is the second commonest causes of renal failure
(b) It is manifestation of poor cardiac output
(c) Responds to frusemide infusion following adequate filling
(d) May be caused by retroperitoneal fibrosis
(e) Leads to acidosis

(a) F (b) T (c) T (d) F (e) T

4. Systemic inflammatory response syndrome criteria includes

(a) Temperature <36°
(b) Heart rate >120
(c) Respiratory rate >20 breaths/min
(d) Reactive protein >5
(e) Haemoglobin <9 gm/dl

(a) T (b) F (c) T (d) F (e) F

5. Following statements regarding oliguria are true

(a) Oliguria is defined as a urinary output <0.5 ml/kg/min
(b) First line of treatment is administration of 20 mg frusemide IV
(c) Urinary osmolality to twice that of plasma then renal failure is present
(d) Metabolic acidosis is identified by blood gas measurements
(e) Serum potassium falls in renal failure

(a) T (b) F (c) T (d) T (e) F

3

Fluid and Electrolyte Acid–Base Balance and Nutrition

Fluid and electrolyte haemostasis is determined by intake and output and is precisely regulated by normal healthy body.

Total body water	=	60% body water (males)
	=	42 litres (70 kg man)
Extracellular fluid	=	14 litres
Intracellular fluid	=	28 litres
Plasma	=	3.5 litres (radioiodinated albumin)

Measurement of ECF volume

A. Evan's blue dye

B. Radioiodine–tracker–thiosulphate

ICF	=	TBW–ECF
Daily water requirement	=	1500 ml/day

Intake ml		*Output ml*	
Liquids	1200	Urine	1500
Solids	1000	Skin	900
Oxidate	300	Faeces	100
Total	2500	**Total**	2500

Water Loss

A. Urine	=	1500 ml/day
B. Insensible losses 37°C for 24 hours	=	0.5 ml/kg/hr
C. Faeces	=	100–200 ml/day
Renal GFR	=	120 ml/min
Loss from ileostomy	=	450 ml
Molarity	=	One mole is a gram mole weight of a substance
Osmolarity	=	Osmosis of a solvent across a semipermeable membrane
1 gm mole	=	6.02×10^{23} molecules
Osmolarity of plasma	=	280–300

Body Compartments

Fluid	*NA⁻*	*K⁻*	*H⁻*	*Cl*	*HCC*	*Protein*	PO_4	SO_4
Plasma	142	45	–	100	25	16	2	1
Intracellular	10	150	–	5	10	60	100	20
Extracellular	144	4		114	30	–	3	3
Gastric juice high	45	30	70	120	25	–	–	–
Gastric juice low	100	45	0.015	115	30	–	–	–
Intestinal juice	120	20	–	110	30	–	–	–
Bile (500–800 ml)	140	5	–	–	40	–	–	–
Pancreatic juice (0.1–0.8)	130	15	–	–	80	–	–	–
Intracellular fluid (0.5–24)	10	150	–	5	10	60	100	20
S fluid	2–10	20–30	–	8–18	30	–	–	–
Colon	60	30	–	40	–	–	–	–

Plasma	=	2(Na + k) + Glucose +Urea
Osmolarity	=	2 × (140 + 4) + 4 + 4
Ex. 0.9	=	58.8 gm __________ 200 mOsm
Dextrose		0.9 __________ 2000 × 0.9/58.5 = 308 (154 +154)
5% Dextrose	=	180 gm __________ 1000 mOsm

$$5\text{ gm} \_\_\_\_\_\_\_\_ \frac{1000}{180} \times 5 = 278$$

Control of Water Intake

Thirst centre in lateral hypothalamus stimulated by

- Plasma osmolarity (>2%)
- Thirst
- ADH
- ECF volume (5–10%)
  - Simulator of arterial Type B
    Receptors–sympathetic stimulator
  - Pressure at renal arterial
    Rennin angiotensin system
  - Na–Renin angiotensin
    Angiotensin
    Vasoconstriction
    ADH
    Aldosterone
    Thirst

Renin Angiotensin System

Stimulated by:

- Pressure at afferent arteriole
  Na at macula densa

- Renin excretion from JG apparatus
  (JG cells, macula densa
- Angiotensinogen
- Angiotensin-I ACE
- Angiotensin-II

Antidiuretic Hormone

- Supraoptic nucleus of posterior pituitary
- Water reabsorption from collecting duct of kidney
- Vasoconstriction in large

ADH	*ADH*
• Plasma osmolarity	• ↑ Plasma osmolarity
• ECF volume	• ↑ ECF volume
• Prolonged exercise	• ↑ Alcohol
• Pain	
• Stress–Surgery/Trauma	

Sodium

Normal: 57 mmol/kg (3900 mmol)
44% ECF
9% ICF
47% bone

- Contributes to major osmolarity of plasma 140 out of 280 (Cl-103, HCO_3-25)
- Upstroke in action potential
- Depolarisation at synapse
  1000 mmol–GI tract, faeces (5 mmol).

Kidney

Plasma Na (136–144 mmol)

PCT 75% ⇨ LH 22% ⇨ DCT 4–5% ⇨ CD 2–3%

Intake: 80–100 mmol/day (5–6 gm)
1–2 mEq/kg/day

HYPERNATREMIA

Causes

Water deficiency: Inadequate intake, environmental and iatrogenic.

Excessive Losses

- Renal losses
- Diabetes insipidus

- Central insipidus
- Central AV deficiency
- Nephrogenic

Extrarenal Losses

- Sweat
- Respiration
- Diarrhoea
- Fever

Excessive Sodium: Intake, Saliva and $NaHCO_3$

Renal failure

Signs/Symptoms

- Mental status changes
- Thirst
- Cardiovascular decomposition
- Edema
- Myoclonus
- Lab measurement
- Weight gain

Management of Hyponatremia

- Decrease inappropriate water loss
- Increase water administration
- Restrict sodium input and increase excretion
- Stop saline and give diuretics
- In hypernatremia water deficit is calculated as:

$$\text{Water deficit } \frac{\text{Observed Na}-140 \times 0.6 \times \text{body weight kg}}{140}$$

TBW = 45 L

Water Excess

- Polydipsia
- Excess of 5% dextrose postoperatively
- Oliguria with normal output
- Addison's disease water load

- SIADH drugs like morphine and barbiturates
- CA Bronchus, CHF and Pneumonia

Clinical Features

Headache, CNS symptoms, nausea, vomiting and coma

Treatment

- Reduce intake
- 1.8% saline
- Treat primary cause

Water Deficit

- Inadequate intake
- Loss of hypotonic fluids

Clinical Features

Thirst, dehydration, oliguria, mental symptoms and coma
treatment
Orally water and 5% dextrose. Treat primary cause
Normal maintenance requirements

Water	0–10 kg	100 ml kg^{-1} daily
	11–20 kg	1000 ml + 50 ml kg^{-1} daily
	21 kg or more	1500 ml + 25 ml kg^{-1} daily

For an adult this is about 30–35 ml kg^{-1} daily
Sodium 1–2 mmol kg^{-1} daily
Potassium 1 mmol kg^{-1} daily

Certain other agents of preoperative fluid therapy include admission of dextrose and insulin to diabetes and setting up a mannitol infusion in patients with obstructive jaundice to reduce the incidence of acute tubular necrosis.

Table 3.1: Loss of body fluids as percentages of body weight

	Adults	*Children (6 months to 6 years of age)*
Mild	4.0	5.0
Moderate	6.0	7.5
Severe	8.0	10.0

Mechanism of Dehydration

TBW = 45 L
ICF (30 L) = ECF (15 L)
30 L = 12 L (1–3 L) (2 L intestinal)
(1 L plasma)

Vomiting	=	2 L losses
Vomiting and dehydration	=	4 L losses
Shock	=	6 L losses
Mild dehydration	=	4% body weight
Moderate dehydration	=	6% body weight
Severe dehydration	=	8% body weight

Methods of Assessing Hyponatremia

a. Measurements of plasma osmolality
b. Plasma level of other electrolytes such as K, Cl, HCO_3 will be low in hyperlipidemia
c. Urine measurements
d. Use or ion selective electrode electrolyte analyser.

In a study by Kennedy and associates in hospital inpatients 41% of cases were iatrogenic caused by diuretics postoperative infusions, 25% related to chest infections and 23% GI or renal salt or water loss.

Management of Hyponatremia

- Revive water and sodium balance and make haemodynamic evaluation and correct underlying cause
- Restrict water intake
- Increase water loss drug, e.g. phenytoin, antagonists
- Increase Na intake hypertonic solutions
- Decrease Na loss
- 50% of deficit + concomitant losses + normal requirement.

Estimation of Na Deficit

Na : 60%
Cl : 20%
HCO_3 : 50%

For example, A 5-years, 90 kg man presents with hypotension, weakness, confusion and oliguria serum Na–120 meg/L

Of fluid	=	8–10% dehydrate × 60% (total body water)
	=	5.4 Litres
Isotonic Na deficit	=	5.4 × 140 = 756 mEq/L
Hypotonic Na deficit	=	(140–120) × 90 × 60 = 1080 meg
	=	½ (1080 + 756) + = 993 meg

HCO_3: 5 mEq/L × 90 × 50% HCO_3 = 225 meg

Patient 24 hour requirement is 5 L of normal saline lamp of $NaHCO_3$ added to each litre.

Potassium is major intracellular cation. Normal plasma–3.5–5.0 mmol/L

Average diet–60–100 mmol

Potassium stimulates release of both insulin and glycogen so that potassium is removed from extracellular fluid

Requirement–1 mEq/kg/day

HYPOKALEMIA

Causes

- Vomiting or nasogastric suction
- Malabsorption
- Diarrhoea
- Laxatic agents
- Ureterosigmoidoscopy
- Fistulae
- Villous papilloma of rectum
- Ion exchange resins
- Renal losses, alkaline
- Megaloblastic anaemia
- Cardiopulmonary anaemia
- Loop diuretic like Frusemide and Thiazides.

Signs/Symptoms

- Muscle cramps
- Loss of tendon reflexes
- Fatigue sleepness
- Tachycardia and hypotension
- Mental abnormality and confusion states
- Cardiac arrhythmias and arrest
- Sensitivity to digitalis

ECG changes include reduction in height of T waves, ST segment depression and occasional T wave inversion.

In severe cases U waves appears, QT interval and QRS interval are widened.

Treatment of Hypokalemia

K deficit = (Normal K–Measurement K)
× 0.4 × body weight in kg

EG; 60 kg females plasma K = 2 mmol/L

K deficit = (4.5–2.0) × 0.4 × 60
= 2.4 × 24 = 60 mmol

Oral Asum

1 tablet–600 mg–8 mmol/K

3–8 tablets/day

Intravenous–20 mmol in each ampule

Not to exceed 10 mmol/hr or 120 mmol/day

In hypokalemia for every $2K^+$ moving from IC to EC compartment $2Na^+$ move inside–extracellular alkalosis and intracellular acidosis.

Hyperkalemia

- Measure K > 5.5 mmol/L
- Medical emergency

Causes

- Haemolysis–mismatched blood transfusions
- Thrombocytosis
- Intake–IV or oral load
- Reduced excretion
- Acute or chronic renal failure
  - Na depletion
  - Steroid deficiency: Addison's disease
  - In appropriate uses of K conserving diuretics
  - Acidosis, diabetes and ketoacidosis
- Ischaemia, chemotherapy and malignant hyperthermia
- Muscle trauma

Signs/Symptoms

Most patients are asymptomatic until plasma K is greater than 6 mmol/L muscle weakness, paralysis, paresthesia, confusion, ileus and loss of tendor reflexes. ECG is best indicator for hyperkalemia

- Tall T waves
- Widened QRS complex
- Wide PR interval

Cardiac arrest may occur in asystole when plasma levels exceed 7 mmol/L.

Treatment

- Stop further potassium
- Insulin 10 U in 50 gm glucose
- $NaHCO_3$: 50 ml of 8.4 % corrects acidosis and returns K to ICF
- Ca gluconate antagonizes the cardiotoxic effect 10 ml of 10% Ca gluconate over 2–3 min is given
- Ion exchange resins, continuous ECG monitoring is required.

Calcium

Body calcium is about 25,000 mmol contained in bone and important for neuromuscular activity

Serum calcium = 2.2–2.5 mmol/L
Normal intake = 1–3 gm/day
Protein bound (50%) Ionized (45%) Bound to other subs (5%)
Acidosis causes ↓ ionized fraction
Alkalosis causes ↓ ionized fraction

HYPOCALCEMIA

Classical symptoms is reduction in plasma ionized calcium concentrate is tetany are with Chvostek's and Trousseau's sign, laryngeal stridor, mental changes and convulsions causes ECG changes are prolongation can be QT interval.

Causes

- Body Metastasis
- Ectopic PTH
- Primary hypoparathyroidism
- Paget's disease of bone
- Prolonged immobilization
- Hypoparathyroidism postsurgical
- Severe pancreatitis
- Renal failure
- Massive blood transfusion
- Sepsis
- Alkalosis

Treatment

- Oxygen by mask patent airway
- 10–20 ml of 10% gluconate slow–IV followed by 40 ml of 10% in 500 ml saline in 4–8 hours.

HYPERCALCEMIA

Signs/Symptoms

- Appears when Ca >3.5 mmol/L
- Depression of CNS, mental, apathy muscle weakness and drowsiness
- Abdominal pain and polyuria metastasis
- Renal calculi ECG ↓ QT interval.

Treatment

- ECF volume expansio–4–6 L of NaCl
- Frusemide–20–40 mg 8 hourly

- Glucocorticoids Ca absorption decrease prednisolone 10–25 mg/day
- Calcitonin and diphosphates bone resorption
- Haemoperitoneal dialysis
- EDTA chelates ionized Ca.

HYPERMAGNESEMIA

- Normal 0.7–0.9 mmol/L
- Renal failure, Mg medication

Signs/Symptoms

Muscle weakness, loss of tendon reflexes, drowness, ↑ P.R. interval, wide QRS, ↑ T.

Treatment

- Dialysis
- Calcium for cardiac arrhythmias
- Induce diuresis 4–6 L saline
- Frusemide 20–40 mg 4–9 hourly.

Hypomagnesemia <1.0 mmol/L

- Prolonged TPN vomiting, diarrhoea
- GI losses: V, D, fistulae
- Alcoholism
- Diuretics
  CL/F: ↓ N–M excitability,
  ECG: ↓ ST,T intervention, ↓ QT

Treatment

Mg chloride or sulphate 30–50 mmol in 1 L of 5% dextrose over 12–24 hours.

HYPOCHLORAEMIA

Causes

- Increased secretion and loss of gastric juice, e.g. in pyloric stenosis and prolonged nasogastric suction
- Increased renal excretion and diuretics
- Disorders of Na regulation–aldosteronism
- Dilution
- Actual hyponatraemia
- Increased bicarbonate retention.

Treatment is that on the underlying cause. An estimate of the chloride deficit may be calculated as follows:

Chloride deficit = (normal plasma chloride (100 mmol 1^{-1})

Measured plasma chloride) × 0.20 × body weight in kg

This is along the lines of estimating Na deficit. If a true chloride deficit exists then it should be replaced with 0.9% NaCl.

HYPERCHLORAEMIA

Causes

- Increased intake of administration
- Decreased production of bicarbonate
- Respiratory alkalosis
- Decreased excretion by the kidney unable to produce bicarbonate, e.g. in renal tubular acidosis
- Dehydration
- Excessive absorption from the gastrointestinal tract, the following uretero-ileostomies.

Treatment is again that of the underlying cause and almost correction of the Na abnormality is of primary importance and may in itself correct the abnormality of chloride.

Normal value

Water = 35 ml/kg × 60 = 2100 ml
Na^+ = 1 mEq/kg × 60 = 60 ml
K^+ = 1 mEq/kg × 60 = 60 ml
Cl = 1.5 mEq/kg × 60 ml = 90 ml
HCO_3 = 0.5 mEq/kg × 60 = 30 ml

Replacement therapy

- Pure gastric loss : 0.45/NaCl + 20–30 mg/KCl/L
- Intestinal juice losses : Ringer lactate + 10 mg/KCl/L
- Third space losses : Ringer lactate or normal saline
- 1st 24 hrs : Na retention
  5% dextrose is fluid of choice
- Urine output of 0.5–1 ml/kg/hour is maintained
- Oliguria urinary Na > 30, B urea > 35, CVP–3–7 cm of water
- Patients of renal failure are to fluid overload. Only insensible losses, blood and fluid losses should be replaced
- After 1st day 1 mmol/kg added as KCl
- Mild surgery : 3–5 ml/kg/hour
- Moderate surgery : 5–7 ml/kg/hour
- Severe : 7–10 ml/kg/hour

Fluid Replacement

Deficit + maintenance + 3rd space losses + op. procedure
Blood loss – Swabs + drapes + suction apparatus + surgical gloves
According body weight

1–10 kg–100 ml/kg for 24 hours
10–20 kg–1000 ml + 20/kg/ for 24 hours
20 kg–1500 ml + 40 ml/kg/ for 24 hours.

Solution Available

Solutions	Na^+	K^+	Cl^-	HCO^3	Ca_2^+	*Uses*
0.9% isotonic	154	–	154	–	–	ECP replacement saline correction of hyponatraemia gastric fluid
0.45% NaCl	77	–	77	–	–	Replacement
Ringer lactate	130	4	109	28	3	Best ECF replacement
5% dextrose	–	–	–	–	–	Correction of insensible losses

Acid-Base Disease

Normal body fluid conc of H^+ ions is 40 mEq/L. Total amount of H^+ ions of 15 L of extracellular body fluid is 600 mEq. Every 3 sec we produce H^+ ions we have buffers and kidney's eliminates 60 mEq of H^+ ions/day. Buffer is an acid–base combination ion which the acid is only partially associated. Buffers system is a weak acid and acid-donating proton H^+. Buffer salt of weak acid or base. Base accepting–a proton H^+

Buffering = Strong acid + buffer
Weak acid + inactive salt
Strong alkali + buffer

To measure arterial blood sample to draw a heparin revised arterial sample (0.05–0.1 ml per ml of blood) from radial artery from wrist and properly iced sample is to be maintained.

Buffers an Acid

A. Plasma
- Bicarbonate
- Plasma protein

B. Red cells
- Bicarbonate–18% of total buffering
- Phosphates

C. Haemoglobin–35%

CO_2 is a byproduct of cellular metabolism and combines with H_2O to produce carbonic acid. There are two pathways to acquire and dispose H^+ ions by the body.

Metabolic pathway–acid from cells–buffered in transit by haemoglobin and eliminated by lungs.

Majority of CO_2 is carried as gas dissolved in water and eliminated as gas and all the other acids are called fixed acids.

PH = Negative algorithm to the base ten of the hydrogen ion combination
= Log[H] = 7.36–7.44
<6.9 – Death

PO_2–measure of dissolved oxygen in plasma–indicates hypoxia

Venous PO_2 : 40

Venous PCO_2 : 45

HCO_3 : 22–28

SaO_2 (oxygen saturation of NB) = Oxy HB × 100/Oxy Hb + Deoxy Hb

SPO_2 = Oxy Hb × 100/Oxy Hb + Deoxy Hb + CO Hb + Meth Hb

Causes of Acidosis

- Increased production of H^+ ion
- Decreased excretion of H^+ ion

Production : Diabetes ketoacidosis (Ketones)
Cellular anoxia (Lactic acid)

Excretion : Renal failure
Respiratory failure

Metabolic Alkalosis

- Renal hyperalimentation
- Secondary hyperaldosteronism
- Exogenous administration of alkaline substances
- Blood transfusion and sodabicarb
- Extrarenal loss of acids like pyloric stenosis.

Respiratory Alkalosis

- Hyperventilation
- Mechanical exercise

ABG Readings

Look at pH

Below 7.35

There is acidosis and then look at PCO_2

PCO_2 above 45 means acidosis is respiratory

- Falls in HCO_3 for 10 mm fall of PCO_2
- Look for increase in HCO_3 for 10 minutes increase in PCO_2 to evaluate
- Below 25 means acidosis is metabolic.

Above 7.45

PCO_2 below 35 means alkalosis is respiratory

- Fall in HCO_3 for 10 mm fall in PCO_2
- Above 45 means alkalosis is metabolic.

Example

1. PCO_2: 40 mm pH 7.25
   Interpretation
   PCO_2 of 40 mm Hg = No respiratory component
   Calculated pH = 7.40
   Measured pH = 7.25
   pH differences = 0.15
   Base deficit = 10 mEq/L = Metabolic acidosis.

Respiratory component: Metabolic acidosis

2. PCO_2–50 mm pH 7.25
   Interpretation
   PCO_2 rise of 10 mm Hg = hypovent + respiratory acidosis
   Calculate pH = 7.30
   Measured pH = 7.25
   pH deficit = 0.05
   Base deficit = 3.33 mEq/L = Metabolic acidosis.

At this stage, we can find out if patient is in acidosis/alkalosis from pH and PCO_2. Find out the exact level of base excess/deficit which needs to be corrected to restore normal acid–base balance. Normal level in mEq/L minus the exported level represents the deficit of bicarbonate and multiple by the no. of litres of extracellular fluid (20% body weight) gives know much of PCO_2 can alter normal. pH. pH–PCO_2 combination gives complete picture.

Method to calculate PCO_2 changes to pH. Each 10 mm Hg PCO_2 produces 0.1 change in pH. If the calculated pH is reasonably close to measured pH, then all the changes are respiratory, If not then there is some metabolic component.

Normal value of buffer base is 50 mEq/L. Bicarbonate is measurement of bicarbonates.

Deficit of Bicarbonate

Normal bicarbonate	= 24 mEq/L
Reported	= 14 mEq/L
Deficit	= 10 mEq
Body weight	= 14 L (20% of 70)
Extracellular deficit of bicarbonate	= 10 × 14 = 140 mEq
Extracellular buffer deficit of older buffers	= 140 + 70 = 210 mEq
Total buffer deficit intracellular	= 420 mEq

Nutritional Support

- An enquiry into amount of weight lost
- History of oral intake
- Prolonged history of vomiting, anorexia or diarrhoea
- Visual assessment of muscle and fat, hair, nails in chronic malnutrition.

Biochemical Assessment

Serum albumin is most commonly available test >3.0 indicates severe malnutrition.

Entral Nutritional Support

- Oral feeding–drug powder 225–250 calories per feed
- Nasoentral tube feeding
- Invasive test feeding.

Parenteral Nutritional Support

Via CVP or via peripheral venous access.

Feeding Solutions

- Kitchen feeds
- Entral formulae
- Polypeptide formulae
- Medium chain triglycerides containing formulae
- Inumunonutrients

Parenteral Feeding

Indications for parenteral feeding

A. Gastrointestinal failures
Prolonged paralytic ileus
Enteric fistulae
Chronic intestinal obstruction
Extensive inflammatory bowel disease
Acute ulceratives colitis

B. To supplement oral feeding in:
Severe burn
Massive or prolonged infection

C. To treat malnutrition preoperatively
Oesophageal carcinoma
Pyloric stenosis

Caloric Values

- Carbohydrates 4 kcal/g
- Protein 4 kcal/g
- Fat 9 kcal/g

Parenteral Solutions

Gastrointestinal failure

- Hypertonic (20% or 50%) dextrose solutions (4 cal/gm)
- Lipid (9 cal/gm)

- MVI and trace elements
- All in one solutions (there in one), amino acids solutions, hypertonic dextrose and lipid emulsions are mixed in single container 100 ml of 25% dextrose + 500 amino acid + 500 ml amino acid + 500 ml normal saline and is the biggest recent adverse in TPN therapy.

Baseline caloric requirement = 28 × body weight in kg

Caloric requirement	% increase
Malnourished patient	+ 10%
Age 18–20 years	+ 10%
Rise in temp	+ 10%
Mobile	+ 10%
Postoperative	+ 15%
Sepsis/Trauma	+ 25%
Burns	+ 35%
Obesity	– 10%
Age >70 years	– 10%
Female sex	– 10%

High increase requirement : Peritonitis, burns

Moderate requirement : Sepsis, trauma

Sample TPN Prescription

Calories

Basal calories	60 × 28	=	1680
For age 18–30 yrs	+10%	=	168
Temp 1°	+10%	=	168
Postoperative status	+15%	=	252
	Total	**=**	**2268**
Protein requirement	60 × 1.5	=	90
Fluid requirement	60 × 40	=	2400
Basal	+10%	=	240
	Total	**=**	**2730 ml**

Electrolyte

Sodium	60 × 1.5	=	90 mEq
Chloride	60 × 1.5	=	90 mEq
Potassium	60 × 1.0	=	60 mEq

Final prescription

Fluid	*Volume*	*Calories*	*Nitrogen*
20% lipid	500 ml	1000	–
10% amino acid	1000 ml	–	12.8
40% dextrose	1000 ml	1200	–
Normal saline	500 ml	–	–
KCl solution	30 ml	–	–
Total	**3030 ml**	**2200**	**12.8**

PROTOCOL USED FOR TPN

Table 3.2: Daily requirements for parenteral nutrition

	Day-I	*Day-II*	*Day-III*	*Day-IV*	*Day-V*
Isolyte P	100 ml/kg	120 ml/kg	130 ml/kg	140 ml/kg	165 ml/kg
25% dextrose or 50%	–	20 ml/kg	30 ml/kg	40 ml/kg	65 ml/kg
Astymin-3	10 ml/kg	15 ml/kg	20 ml/kg	30 ml/kg	40 ml/kg
MVI	1 ml	1 ml	1 ml	1 ml	1 ml
KCl	1 ml/kg	1 ml/kg	1 ml/kg	1 ml/kg	1 ml/kg
Fluid and calorie					
Fluid ml/kg	112 ml	157 ml	182 ml	212 ml	272 ml
Calories	22	47	60	74	10

Fluid Replacement

Maintenance 1500 ml + 20 ml/kg body weight in excess of 20 kg
Replacement of other losses (e.g. nasogastric tube, drains, etc.).

Protein requirement

1.0–1.2 g/kg/day

Energy requirement

33 cal/kg/day

19–20 cal/kg/day in diabetic and obese patients; 20%–30% of calories from lipids and 70%–80% from carbohydrates. In patients with respiratory failure the lipid component should be higher.

Standard multivitamins and electrolytes

Sodium (mEq)	70–120
Potassium (mEq)	41.5–103
Phosphate (mmol)	15–30
Calcium (mEq)	8.12–16.24
Multivitamins	10 ml daily
Vitamin K	10 mg every week subcutaneously
Trace elements	1–3 ml after 7 days

Table 3.3: Composition of some commercial formulations of parenteral nutrition available in India

Formulation	*Clinomel NS-800*	*Clinimix N9G20E*	*Kabiven*	*Vitrimix*	*Calemix-G*
Volume (L)	2	2	2	1	1
Nitrogen (g)	9.3	9.1	10.8	7	9.6
Total calories	1825	2020	1900	1000	1040
Non-protein calories	1600	1800	1600	800	800
Glucose (calories)	800	800	800	300	350
Lipid (calories)	800	1000	800	500	450
Sodium (mmol)	56	70	64	38	27
Potassium (mmol)	48	60	48	15	1.5
Magnesium (mmol)	4	5	8	1.1	1.5
Calcium (mmol)	3.6	4.5	4	1.9	Na
Phosphate (mmol)	24	30	20	Na	5.4
Acetate (mmol)	100	100	78	Na	61
Chloride (mmol)	64	80	93	37	35
pH	6	6	5.6	5.2	5.6–6.4
Osmolarity (mOsm)	1020	840	1060	1130	1110
Remarks	3-in-1	Lipid added separately	3-in-1	PPN	PPN

PPN = Peripheral Parenteral Nutrition

QUESTIONS AND ANSWERS

1. **In order to understand fluid balance, you must appreciate normality. In the standard 70 kg man how is the sum up of fluid input(s) versus output(s)? Express these in two columns of figures which must tally.**

Oral fluid	2,000 ml
Water of metabolism ($CHO \rightarrow CO_2 + H_2O$)	500 ml
	2,500 ml
Output per day	
Urine	1,500 ml
Faeces	400 ml
Insensible losses	600 ml
	2,500 ml

2. **Which group of people in the hospital are probably the best suited to setting up really difficult i.v. drips?**

   Ans:

   Adults: The anaesthetists (especially those in ICU). Setting up i.v. drips under adverse conditions is major part is their skill.

   Babies: Either the paediatrician of paediatric anaesthetist

3. **Outline a standard intravenous fluid regime for the first 24 hours after a trouble-free partial gastrectomy that did require blood transfusion.**

   Ans:

3,000 ml of fluid	:	2,000 ml is the bare minimum
	:	1,000 ml extra is added to counteract preoperative starvation and losses from the swabs, evaporation, etc.

   50 mmol Na^+

   30–50 mmol K^+

   1,000 ml dextrose saline + 10 mmol KCl 8 hourly

   Or

   1,000 ml 5% dextrose + 5 mmol KCl in 8 hours
   500 ml normal saline + 5 mmol KCl in 4 hours
   500 ml 5% dextrose + 5 mmol KCl in 4 hours
   1,000 ml 5% dextrose + 10 mmol KCl in 8 hours

   Each regime gives the same quantities of water, K^+, N^+, but the former is far less wasteful of nursing time.

4. **What time of day are urinary catheters traditionally removed and why?**

   Ans: First thing in the morning voids (e.g. 500 a.m) and never at week-ends

   Reason: If the patient voids spontaneously there is no problem

   If retension recurs, this will be by the afternoon when staff are available to assess it, and perhaps recatheterize.

   Catheter removals at other time cause severe logistic upsets.

5. **How do you interpret these postoperative figures in a 20-year-old patient explored for a ruptured spleen and found to have merely aminor mesenteric bruise–Hb 11 g, Urea 3, Na 119, K 3.1, HCO_2 20? What intravenous regime would you advise?**

   Ans: Overhydration: The patient was probably regarded as having intraperitoneal bleeding and 1–2 litres of clear fluid before it became apparent that the injury was trivial.

   Intravenous regime: Limit fluid (e.g. 1,500 ml D-saline + 25 mmol KCl/24 hours) and allow the patient's metabolism to sort itself out.

6. **Does the usual management of hypokalaemia differ from that of hyponatraemia?**

   Ans: Yes, remember that these figures are concentrations and are not absolute values.

   Low K^+ Concentration is usually due to loss of K^+ supplement

   Low Na^+ concentration is usually due to excess water

   RX–fluid restriction (hypertonic saline is a dangerous fluid. It tends to push elderly patients into heart failure and needs to be used only very rarely).

7. **What is the hepatorenal syndrome? Is it important in surgery? What standard steps are taken to prevent it?**

   Ans: Hepatorenal syndrome is the association of severe renal failure with liver failure, i.e. jaundice.

   Acute oliguria and uraemia is the major cause of death in jaundiced patients undergoing large operations. Prevention is by:

   a. Ensuring adequate hydration with no episode of hypotension
   b. Catheter to ensure measurement of urinary output

c. Mannitol induced osmotic diuresis before, during and after operation to retain an adequate urinary output (>30 ml)/hr) and thus 'protect' the kidneys.
Use of the regime has virtually eliminated the postoperative hepatorenal syndrome.

8. The average daily water balance in a healthy adult in a temperate climate indicate
(a) An intake of 1,000 ml of water from solid food
(b) 150 ml from oxidation
(c) A loss of 400 ml from expired air
(d) A loss of least 600 ml from insensible cutaneous losses
(e) A faecal loss of 350 ml

Ans: (a) T (b) F (c) T (d) T (e) T

Water intake is derived from solid food which accounts for 1,000 ml per day and beverages which account for 1200 ml per day. Water produced from oxidation accounts for approximately 300 ml per day. Water loss includes 1500 ml of urine output, approximately 1,000 ml of insensible loss from the skin and lungs and a further 100 ml in the faeces.

9. Metabolic alkalosis
(a) May be caused by Cushing's syndrome
(b) May produce Cheyne-Stokes respiration
(c) Produces renal epithelial damage
(d) Produces intracellular alkalosis
(e) May be caused by ureterosigmoidostomy

Ans: (a) T (b) T (c) T (d) F (e) F

Metabolic alkalosis is characterized by a primary increase in the plasma bicarbonate concentration with a consequent decrease in hydrogen ion concentration. By definition it is caused by a non-respiratory cause and often persists after the primary cause is removed. The cause may be due to loss of unbuffered hydrogen ion which can be of gastrointestinal original, e.g. gastric aspiration, vomiting with pyloric stenosis, or chloride losing diarrhea. The renal causes of hydrogen ion loss include mineralocorticoid excess (e.g. Cushing's syndrome and Conn's syndrome), potassium depletion and drugs with mineralocorticoid activity (e.g. carbon oxalone). Alkalosis may cause secondary renal injury.

10. The indications for pulmonary arterial catheterization are
(a) Ventricular auerysm
(b) Ischaemia related subaortic valve stenosis
(c) Surgery for dissecting abdominal aneurysm
(d) Severe pulmonary disease
(e) Frequent arterial blood sampling

Ans: (a) T (b) T (c) T (d) T (e) F

The indications for the insertion of a pulmonary artery catheter include established or anticipated left ventricular dysfunction (e.g. valvular heart disease, ventricular aneurysm, recent myocardial infarction, etc.), aortic surgery requiring cross clamping of the vessel (e.g. thoracoabdominal aortic dissection repair) and severe pulmonary disease (e.g. pulmonary hypertension, pulmonary emboli).

11. The assessment of the malnourished patient
(a) Does not include dynamometric studies
(b) May involve a lymphocyte count

(c) Includes serum transferrin assays
(d) Reveals a positive candida skin test
(e) Is confirmed by a body mass index of 25

Ans: (a) F (b) T (c) T (d) F (e) F

The assessment of patient who require nutritional support involves a dietary history and clinical examination including height and weight for calculation of the body. Mass index (normal range is 20–24.9). Special investigations available are biochemical (albumin and transferrin), immunological (delayed type sensitivity), anthropometric (triceps skin fold thickness) and dynamometric (hand grip strength).

12. The daily nutritional requirement in a 70 kg man are

(a) 4 g/kg of nitrogen
(b) 90 mg of vitamin C per day
(c) Half a litre of normal saline to satisfy the Na^+ requirement
(d) Increased by 61% in head injury patients
(e) Increased by aspirin

Ans: (a) F (b) F (c) T (d) T (e) T

The daily nutritional requirement of a 70 kg include 14 g of nitrogen, 70 mmol of sodium per day and 50 mg of vitamin C per day. Certain clinical conditions require supplementation, e.g. sepsis, ileus, pancreatitis, ulcerative colitis, multiple trauma, renal failure and liver disease. Drugs such as aspirin may also increase requirements.

4

Haemorrhage

HAEMORRHAGE, CLOTTING DISORDERS AND BLOOD PRODUCTS

Arterial haemorrhage	:	Bright, red, spurt
Venous haemorrhage	:	Dark, red, steady
Primary haemorrhage	:	At time of operation or injury
Reactionary	:	May follow primary haemorrhage within 24 hours (usually 5–6 hours)
Secondary haemorrhage	:	4–14 days at time of infection
External haemorrhage	:	Revealed
Internal haemorrhage	:	Concealed
Arterial haemorrhage	:	Bright, red, spurt
Venous haemorrhage	:	Dark, red, steady

MEASURING BLOOD LOSS

Infant	:	80–85 ml/kg
Adult	:	65–70 ml/kg
Blood clot	:	500 ml
Closed fracture	:	500–1500 ml
Swab weighting	:	(1 g/ml)

Swab × 1.5 for blood loss

Prolonged surgery	:	Total swab measurement × 2
Hemoglobin level	:	12–16 gm/dl

Blood is stored at 4°C and rapid transfusion can cause arrhythmias and intraoperative hypothermia, cellular metabolism, membrane ion pump failure, haemolysis leading to hyperkalemia and acidaemia. Anticoagulant (citrate to chelate Ca), loss of clotting factors and active platelets result in coagulopathy during massive transfusion.

TREATMENT OF HAEMORRHAGE

- Pressure and packing
- Position and rest, e.g. elevation
- Catching of active bleeders and drainage and suturing
- Blood transfusion

CLOTTING FACTORS, USE OF BLOOD PRODUCTS AND BLOOD TRANSFUSIONS

1. Clotting disorders
2. Screening
3. History of previous bleeding problems
4. Platelet count, prothrombin time.

CAUSES OF SURGICAL BLEEDING PARTIAL THROMBOPLASTIN TIME (PTT)

1. Acquired bleeding disorders
2. Shock and extensive trauma
3. Rapid transfusion
4. Postoperative bleeding due to inadequate haemostasis
5. Secondary fibrinolysis
6. DIC.

Bleeding time: Actual prolonged bleeding is associated with platelet aggregation disorders.

Thrombin time: Evaluates fibrinogen to fibrin conversion with thrombin used to evaluate DIC and chronic liver disease.

Clotting factor for ref. such as type A hemophilia and von Willebrand's.

Blood Replacement

a. Crystalloid can be used to replace blood, an initial ratio of 3 ml of crystalloid to each 1 ml of blood lost. As the volume increases the ratio must increase because of fall in plasma ratio when colloid, packed cells and red blood cells is administered the ratio is 1:1.
b. Blood group and type must be matched including ABO group and RH factors.
c. Tests for hepatitis, HIV, CMV should be mandatory alone.

Blood Products

A. Fresh frozen plasma

1. As a replacement of coagulation factors.
2. Can be used to reverse the effects of Coumadin as it replaces I, VII, IX, X.
3. Can be used in nonspecific manner, not requiring cross-matching.

B. Cryoprecipitate

1. Measures 5 to 30 ml in single plastic bag, rich in factor VIII, fibrinogen and fibronectin.
2. Useful in treatment of hemophilia A and von Willebrand's disease.

C. Factor VIII concentrates

1. Useful in treating hemophilia A
2. Risk of hepatitis is more

Human Albumin 4.5%

Rich in protein stored at 4°C suitable following protein loss, e.g. Burns.

Fibrinogen

Used in patients of sense depletion of fibrinogen, e.g. DIC and congenital afibrogenemia.

Packed Cell Volume

Patients of chronic anemia, transfusion therapy. Good Packing by letting blood sediment and removing plasma or centrifugations of whole blood at 2000 gm for 15–20 minutes.

Platelet Concentrate

Transfusion to patient with thrombocytopenia prepared by centrifugation of platelet rich plasma at 1200–1500 g for 15–20 minutes.

Blood Stored

Blood is stored at 4°C ± 20°C. It is allowed to stand higher temperature for more than 2 hours. CPD blood has a shelf-life of 5 weeks, but RBC suffer temporary reduction in sugar transfer (24–72 hours) and should be transferred within 7 days, WBC and VII, V platelets are considerably reduced in stored blood.

Position of IC Fluids

	Na	*K*	*Cl*	*HCO_3*	*Lactate*
Plasma	137–147	4–5.5	95–105	22–25	–
1/5 isotonic saline	153	–	153	–	–
4.3/dextrose	30.6	–	30.6	–	–
1/5 isotonic saline	–	–	–	–	–
Ringer lactate	30	4	110	28	–

CVP Measurement

Saline manometer used for measuring central nervous pressure. Zero reference point at midaxillary level and normal is 5–8 cm.

Autotransfusion

Restoring patient's blood volume by transfusion by own blood by autotransfusion apparatus. For elective surgery patient may donate his own blood 3 weeks prior to operations.

Complications of Transfusion

A. Immunologic transfusion reaction include:
   1. Haemolytic transfusion reaction
   2. Febrile transfusion reaction
   3. Post-transfusion thrombocytopenia
   4. Anaphylactic shock

5. Urticaria
6. Graft Vs host disease.

Symptoms of haemolytic reaction include fever, constrictive sensation of chest, pain in lumbar region, hypotension, haemoglobinuria, bleeding due to DIC and renal failure.

Management

1. O_2 inhalation
2. Stop transfusion
3. Blood samples to be checked
4. Antibiotics
5. Investigations for DIC
6. Management of hypotension with volume expanders, ringer lactate, vasoactive drugs and good renal function maintained a diuretic therapy.

QUESTIONS AND ANSWERS

True or False

1. The prothrombin time is prolonged in

(a) Haemophilia F
(b) Haemolytic Jaundice F
(c) Vitamin K deficiency T
(d) Gall stone obstructing common bile duct T
(e) Patients given heparin F

2. Complications of blood transfusion include

(a) Refractory platelet function T
(b) Urticaria T
(c) Fat embolism F
(d) Brucellosis T
(e) Immunosuppression T

3. Macrocystic anaemia follows

(a) Radical gastrectomy T
(b) Jejunal diverticulae F
(c) Crohn's disease T
(d) Pregnancy T
(e) Anticonvulsant therapy T

4. The following statements regarding plasma substitutes are true

(a) Gelofusine and haemocoel are physiologically the closest the plasma T
(b) Hartmann's solution contains 5 mmol/L of potassium F
(c) 5% dextrose solution contains no sodium T
(d) Cell saver techniques are passive reinfusion of lost blood T
(e) Normal saline has a pH of 8 T

5. **Disseminated intravascular coagulation**
   - (a) Platelet fibrin thrombi cause organ ischaemia — T
   - (b) Blood found in sputum — T
   - (c) Follow massive blood transfusion — T
   - (d) Require anticoagulation — T
   - (e) Is associated and subarachnoid — T
6. **Baskett's classification of shock (1991)**
   - (a) Septicaemia is described as invasive shock — F
   - (b) Loss of 3 liters of blood is grade 4 — T
   - (c) There is no change in respiratory rate following loss of 25% blood volume — F
   - (d) Pulse pressure is increased in stage 3 — F
   - (e) Capillary refill is normal until 15% of blood volume lost — T
7. **What is a transfusion reaction? How would you know your patient was having one? What action should you take to treat the patient and diagnose the cause?**

   Ans.: Transfusion reaction is immunological response by recipient to incompatible blood. There may be minor pyrogenic reaction to components of compatible blood. Sudden spurts of pyrexia, rigors, rash, backache, tachycardia may proceed to bronchospasm, angio-neurotic oedema, anaphylaxis and death.

   A major ABO mismatch produces complete vasomotor collapse.

   Treatment: Remove blood and replace with saline and new set. Antihistamine (chlor-pheniramine 25 mg IV), (Hydrocortisone 100 mg IV), Adrenaline 0 to 0.5 ml slowly. Inform blood bank; send then the suspected blood and giving set; a new specimen of clotted and urine sample.
8. **What is commonest cause of mismatched blood transfusion?**

   Ans.: Chemical error in labeling of the donor blood either at venesection or in the laboratory or at recipient's bedside.
9. **What are the lowest level of platelets usually regard as adequate in patient about to undergo a routine major surgical operation?**

   Ans.: (100,000 mm^3); below this are risks of bleeding, transfusion and operation.
10. **What are main features of acute DIC?**

    Ans.: Haemorrhage, mostly from oozing from venepuncture and surgical sites followed by circulatory collapse, cerebral coma, anaemia.
11. **Where would you find splenunculi at operation?**

    Ans.: Near the hilum of spleen, omentum, pelvis, lesser sac.
12. **What is clinical symptoms and treatment of transfusion reaction?**

    Ans.: Clinical: New bottle of blood recently put up. Relatively sudden (5–30 mins) onset of pyrexia, rigors, backache ± rash, tachycardia. May proceed (rarely) via bronchospasm → angioneurotic oedema → (even more rarely) anaphylaxis → death. A major ABO mismatch produces complete vasomotor collapse.

    Treatment: Remove blood + given set, and replace with saline and new set. Antihistamine (e.g. Chlorpheniramine 25 mg IV). Hydrocortisone 100 mg IV (Adrenaline). 1:1000 IM 0–5 ml. slowly) analgesics.
13. **What is the commonest cause of a mismatched blood transfusion?**

    Clerical error in the labelling of the donor blood either at venesection, in the laboratory or at the recipient's bedside. This account for 3/4 of all mismatches.

14. What are the main features of gross acute disseminated intravascular coagulation?

Haemorrhage–often first noticed as persistent oozing from venepuncture sites and surgical incisions. Circulatory collapse ± multiple microthrombicerebral, convulsions. Renal oliguria, (Anuria the thrombotic complications may also sometimes occur on their own).

15. Where might you expect to find splenunculi at operation?

Near the hilum of the spleen; in the omentum, occasionally elsewhere. If retained after therapeutic splenectomy, they may hypertrophy and restore some splenic function.

16. The prothrombin time is prolonged in

(a) Haemophilia
(b) Haemolytic jaundice
(c) Vitamin K deficiency
(d) Gallstones obstructing the common bile duct
(e) Patients given heparin

Ans.: (a) F (b) F (c) T (d) T (e) F

The prothrombin time measures the extrinsic pathway of coagulation, involving factors VII and X, but not factor VIII which is responsible for haemophilia. The vitamin K dependent factors, III, V, VII, IX and X prolong the PT if deficiency. Diseases affecting liver function such as cholestasis will also interfere with the coagulation cascade. Clotting may also be affected by drugs such as heparin and warfarin. Warfarin is a vitamin K antagonist whilst heparin increases complex formation between anti-thrombin III and activated serum protease factors (thrombin, XIIa, XIa, Xa, IXa, VIIa).

17. Complications of blood transfusions include

(a) Refractory platelet function
(b) Urticaria
(c) Fat embolus
(d) Brucellosis
(e) Immunosuppression

Ans.: (a) T (a) T (c) F (d) T (e) T

Other systemic complications are anaphylaxis, volume overload, hypothermia, hyperkalaemia, acidosis, transmission of hepatitis, and HIV. Anaphylaxis is invariably due to a clerical error and leads to a transfusion of incompatible blood.

18. Macrocytic anaemia follows

(a) Radical gastrectomy
(b) Jejunal diverticulae
(c) Crohn's disease
(d) Pregnancy
(e) Anticonvulsant therapy

(a) T (b) F (c) T (d) T (e) T

Macrocytic anaemia is the result of vitamin B_{12} deficiency. Malabsorption of this vitamin follows total gastrectomy due to the loss of intrinsic factor. Deficiency of B_{12} may also be due to impaired absorption of the vitamin in the terminal ileum, e.g. Crohn's disease. The requirements increase during pregnancy.

19. The following statements regarding plasma substitutes are true

(a) Gelofusine and haemocoel are physiologically the closest to plasma
(b) Hartmann's solution contains 5 mmol/L of potassium
(c) 5% dextrose solution contains no sodium

(d) Cell saver techniques are passive reinfusions of lost blood
(e) Normal saline has a pH of 8

(a) F (b) T (c) T (d) F (e) F

The fluid replacement that most closely resembles plasma is Hartmann's solution. Gelofusine and haemocoel are colloids which lack electrolytes. 5% dextrose in an isotonic fluid replacement containing water and an isomer of glucose. Blood salvage involves low pressure aspiration followed by filtration or centrifugation prior to reinfusion into the patient. It is suitable in operation where large blood volumes may be lost in the absence of faecal contamination or malignancy, e.g. cardiac surgery, hepatic surgery.

20. Disseminated intravascular coagulation

(a) Platelet fibrin thrombi cause end organ ischaemia
(b) Blood is found in the sputum
(c) Follow massive blood transfusion
(d) Requires anticoagulation
(e) Is associated with subarachnoid haemorrhage

Ans.: (a) T (b) F (c) T (d) F (e) T

DIC is the inappropriate activation of coagulation with the production of platelet fibrin thrombi, fibrin degradation products and depletion of coagulation factors. The complication of haemorrhage and end-organ ischaemia requires immediate support measures. Subarachnoid haemorrhage, retroperitoneal haemorrhage and renal failure are associated complications. Management requires replacement of coagulation factors, organ support and treatment of the underlying causes in the intensive care setting.

21. What do you assess shock?

(a) Assess veins, low central venous pressure (CVP), and a history of fluid loss, trauma, surgery, resuscitation begins with fluid challenge. The volume given should be based on an estimated of the patient's weight. Ringer's lactate (30 ml/kg) should be infused rapidly.
(b) If neck veins are distended, CVP in increased, or arrhythmia is present, a cardiac cause must be considered.
(c) If shock persists, a pulmonary artery line (Swan-Ganz catheter) should be inserted.
(d) Treatment of arrhythmia is followed by consideration of a pacemaker and long-term pharmacologic support.
(e) Causes of low or normal filling pressures includes severe hypovolemia, sepsis, severe trauma, and neurogenic shock.

22. How do assess cardiac tamponade and move?

(a) High filling pressures and poor cardiac function suggest several compressive causes. Mechanical causes should be considered and treated early. This may require pericardiocentesis for treatment of tamponade and pericarditis, ventilation for support of patients with pulmonary embolism, and surgery for some cardiac problems. Therapy for the failing heart is directed at offloading the intravascular space by diuresis. Subsequent therapy is more specific to the pattern of cardiac failure. During resuscitation, constant monitoring of the level of oxygenation and acid-base balance is necessary. The use of nitrates for vasodilation is based on the combined cardiac assessment.

(b) Cardiac tamponade occurs in a wide variety of clinical scenarios, including trauma, postoperative states, tuberculosis, tumors, aortic dissection, uraemia and anticoagulation. The hallmark of cardiac tamponade is equalization of cardiac pressure in all four chambers. Whereas tamponade can be confused with left ventricular failure, noninvasive cardiac testing is diagnostic.

23. What is significance SVR and management of check?

(a) If the systemic vascular resistance (SVR) is high and the cardiac output (CO) is low, the patient is Hypovolemic and needs volume expansion with attention to acidosis. Be prepared for continued fluid for third space losses. Treat the cause of blood or fluid loss.

(b) With low SVR, the diagnostic possibilities are treatment aims to remove the cause of shock, provide fluids (balanced crystalloids), and optimize electrolytes and acid-base balance. Renal dose dopamine may help to preserve renal function. If CO is very low, use Dobutamine, 5 µg/kg/min. Alpha-adrenergic agents should be used to provide vasoconstriction only after other therapy fails. Start vasoconstrictive therapy using phenylephrine, 100 µg, to increase resistance, or use norepinephrine starting at 0.01 µg/kg/min. Monitor organ function and peripheral circulation closely.

Flow Chart: Haemorrhage

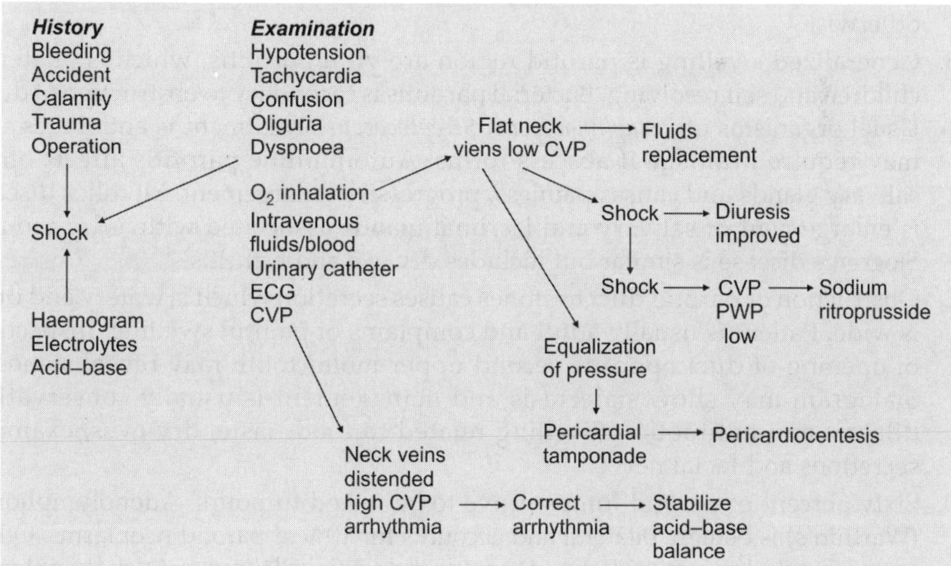

5 Head and Neck/ Lymphadenopathy

LUMPS

A. Early step in the diagnosis of lumps in the head and neck is to decide whether lump is in skin or deep. If lump is deep you will have to decide which anatomical region it belongs and relation to sternomastoid muscle. The anatomical regions are pretracheal, anterior and posterior triangles.

B. Cervical auricle is an accessory ear lobe and situated low in neck anterior to sternomastoid. Treatment is by cosmetic removal.

C. Other swelling such as sebaceous cyst, dermoid, lipomas, fibromas, basal and squamous cell carcinomas has been dealt. Parotid gland is largest parotid gland situated below acoustic meatus between mandible and sternomastoid muscle Superficial 80%, Deep 20%.

LUMPS IN PAROTID REGION

A. Parotid region swelling if it is deep to skin then it is the parotid gland until proved otherwise.

B. Generalized swelling is parotid region are viral parotitis, which is bilateral, children and self resolving. Bacterial parotitis is secondary to obstruction of duct. Usual organisms are *Staphylococcus, Streptococcus*. Treatment is antibiotics and may require drainage if abscess forms. Autoimmune parotitis affects other salivary glands and causes painless, progressive enlargement. Mikulicz disease is enlargement of salivary and lacrimal glands associated with a dry mouth. Sjogren's disease is similar but includes dry eye and arthritis.

C. Obstruction of parotid duct to stones causes secretion which is watery and duct is wide. Patient is usually adult and complains of painful swelling. Inspection of opening of duct opposite second upper molar tooth may reveal stenosis. Sialogram may show sialectasis and management is usually conservative dilators and antibiotics. Swelling related to food, taste, dry eyes, examine secretions and facial nerve.

D. Sixty percent of parotid lumps prove to be mixed tumours. Adenolymphoma (Warthin's) is benign, bilateral and accounts for 10% of parotid neoplasms. Other tumours include mucoepidermoid tumour and acinic cell tumour. Adenolymphoma occurs in parotid lower pole present as smooth older cystic, fluctuant swelling. Treatment is superficial parotidectomy. Adenolymphoma occurs in parotid gland as smooth swelling in older men. It produces hot spot in technetium. Pleomorphic adenoma 80%, common, histologically shows epithelial cells, myoepithelial cells. It is unilateral, painless, firm, slow growing swelling. Malignancy in salivary gland is nodular. Diagnosis is by FNAC, CT scan treatment is excision.

If nodes are involved block dissection of neck is done.

TNM staging

T1 Tumor <2 cm
T2 2–4 cm
T3 4–6 cm
T4 >6 cm
N1 Ipsilateral
N2 3–6 cm
N3 >6 cm nodes
M1 Metastasis

Radical parotidectomy is done which includes removal of both lobes of parotid mandible, facial nerve.

E. The most common non-neoplastic solitary nodule in parotid region is cyst.
F. Mixed tumours contains adenoma cells surrounded by mucin. It is important for performing a formal superficial parotidectomy as these incompletely encapsulated tumours have high degree of local recurrence. In superficial parotidectomy incision is made anterior to ear and S shaped curve in upper neck. Facial nerve trunk is identified and all tissue superior to it has to be excised with the tumour.
G. Malignancy in salivary gland is hard, nodular diagnosis is by FNAC, CT scan. Treatment is excision. It lymph nodes are involved block dissection of neck is done.

LUMPS IN ANTERIOR TRIANGLE OF NECK

A. It lies below the digastrics and in front of sternomastoid. Branchial sinus present as tiny hole in lower part of neck and tract runs up the neck and develops of second arch does not close branchial cleft. Patient is a child, opening is in front of anterior border of sternomastoid and treatment of excision of whole tract. Branchial cysts emerge under anterior border of sternomastoid Age <20.
B. Branchial cysts is formed by squamous cell inclusions and appears as swelling and sometimes abscess and lies deep to sternomastoid muscle with fluctuation and no transillumination. Treatment is excision.
C. Carotid body tumour is chemodectoma arising from cells in carotid body grows slowly. Histological it is a new chromaffin paraganglioma. Lump is hard, pulsatile at carotid, bifurcation, beneath the anterior border to sternomastoid, mobile form side-to-side and not up and down. MRI and carotid angiography are helpful in diagnosis and removal is excision by excision by giving vertical incision.
D. Pharyngeal pouch is pulsion diverticulum as obstruction at cricopharyngeus muscle in GERD patients and mucosa produces through Kellian's dehiscence. Elderly males complain that first mouthful is easily swallowed but subsequent obstructs in upper oesophagus. Patient complains of dysphagia, regurgitation at night and pouch is demonstrated or barium swallow and treatment is excision

mucosal pouch excised and closed. Laryngoceles are painless. There can be external, internal and may be associated above anterior belly of digastrics.

LUMPS IN SUBMANDIBULAR GLAND

A. Submandibular salivary gland measures about 3–4 cm situated beneath angle of jaw. Its superficial portion is outside mylohyoid muscle and deep is below it lies in floor of mouth. Its duct opens in floor of mouth.

B. Generalized enlargement of submandibular gland is secondary to stone formation localized enlargement has same aetiology as parotid, less common and greater portion is malignant. It can be sialadenitis, stone and tumor as secretions are viscous and duct narrower, stone formation with subsequent secondary infection with staphylococcus. It causes swelling and oedema of floor of mouth causing respiratory obstruction (Ludwig's angina). Condition can occur at any edge, common in young adult, intermittent painful swelling in mouth. Stone may be palpable in duct in the floor of mouth beneath the tongue. Stones are radioopaque and sialogram will delineate submandibular duct in floor of mouth. Submandibular gland is removed by giving 2.5 cm incision below angle of jaw. Deep portion can be removed after protecting lingual and hypoglossal nerves.

C. *Posterior triangle:* (Behind sternomastoid, in front of trapezius, above clavicle). If there are many small lumps, think of nodes–TB or viruses such as HIV or EBC (infectious mononucleosis) or, if over 20 years, consider lymphoma or metastases. Cervical ribs may intrude into this area.

D. *Tests:* Ultrasound shows lump consistency, CT defines masses in relation to their anatomical neighbors. Do virology and Mantoux test. CXR may show malignancy or reveal bilateral hilar lymphadenopathy; here you should consider sarcoid. Consider fine-needle aspiration (FNAC).

Table 5.1: Cervical lymph nodes and their areas of drainage

	Name	*Area of drainage*
1.	Submental group	Tip of tongue, anterior end of lower lip, floor or mouth and lower gum, bilateral drainage.
2.	Submandibular group	Centre of forehead, nose, paranasal sinuses, front of neck, lips, anterior two-thirds of tongue.
3.	Buccal and mandibular group	Cheek, lower eyelid
4.	Preauricular group	Temple, vertex, eyelids, orbit, external acoustic meatus
5.	Occipital group	Back of scalp, posterior edge of pinna
6.	Supraclavicular group	Occipital nodes, axillary nodes, breast, body wall
7.	Infraclavicular group	Lower neck, preaxial border of upper limb, body wall, breast
A.	Tonsillar node (anterosuperior deep cervical node)	Subcutaneous nodes, tonsil
B.	Jugulo-omohyoid node (posteroinferior deep cervical node)	Submental group, submandibular group, posterior third of the tongue. These nodes, therefore, receive all the lymph drainage

CONDITION OF MOUTH

A. Cleft lip and palate

1. Cleft lip 2nd commonest congenital anomaly after club foot 1:750. 75% unilateral. Failure of fusion of facial processes.
2. Cleft palate has problems with speech (velopharyngeal closure) vowels feeding as inability to suck, infection. Cleft lip repaired at Millard's rule of 10 weeks of age, 10 pounds of weight, 10 gm% haemoglobin. Treatment is irregular flap repair (Tennyson's Randall) or Millard's rotation advancement technique.

   Cleft palate is repaired before 12–18 months of age below child starts to speak and not before 6 months surgical treatment is Veau-Wardill Kilner (V-Y) double reversing plasty and Langenbeck operation.
3. Mucous retention cyst develops when a duct of mucous gland becomes blocked are usually in lower lip or buccal mucous and treatment is excision.
4. Ranula is unilateral cystic swelling in floor of mouth formed from blocked mucous gland and accessory salivary gland. Patents are swelling to semitransparent, grey, cystic transilluminates.

   They may plunge into neck. Treatment is excision or marsupalization.
5. Dermoid cyst are midline swelling on floor of mouth origination from ectoderm usually present painless cystic or putty like swelling treatment is excision.
6. Development cyst same as dermoid cyst but occurs in bone and commonest is globular maxillary cyst and treatment is excision.
7. Dental cyst develops from enamel or root as erupted or decayed tooth. It usually present as painless swelling, diagnosis is by X-ray and treatment is excision.
8. Dentigerous cyst contains unerupted tooth develop around upper or lower third molar with painful swelling. Diagnosis is by X-ray and treatment is excision.
9. Alveolar abscess is formed in root of decaying tooth, tracts down of forms abscess beneath cheek or mandible. Child present with swelling and throbbing ache of jaw. Treatment is excision.
10. Benign tumors of mouth include epulis which is localized swelling of gum. These may be fibrous, bony, granulomatous.
    a. Admantinoma is locally invasive tumor derived from enamel responsible for basal cell carcinoma. It is multiloculated painless swelling of jaw. These are egg shell cracking over overlying bone, X-ray shows honeycomb appearance and local curettage and excision is done.
    b. Carcinoma of lip is called countryman's lip is keratinizing squamous cell carcinoma, 93% occur in lower lip and drain to submental nodes. Ulcer has a raised rolled edge treated with surgery or radiotherapy. Surgery is wedge resection.
    c. Squamous cell carcinoma and malignant melanoma are rare.

LUMPS IN POSTERIOR TRIANGLE

A. *Cervical rib*
   1. In 1 in 200 people, the costal element of seventh cervical vertebra overdevelops. It is bony, attached to first normal rib, and may be fibrous strand. Patient notices swelling or tenderness in neck on effected side. A cervical rib causing neurological symptoms may be managed conservatively with physiotherapy. A cervical rib causing vascular neurological problems should be excised.

B. *Cervical lymphadenopathy*
   1. Swelling in neck clinically
   2. Screening test also include full blood count, ESR, X-ray chest, open biopsy and excision in done acute inflammatory lymphadenopathy treatment is antibiotics and drainage. Treatment of tubercular lymphadenopathy is anti-tubercular drugs followed by excision.
   3. Malignant lymphoma are neoplasm of Hodgkin's disease and non-Hodgkin's lymphoma. Symptom typically present as lymphadenopathy, fever, weight loss and night sweats.

      Stage-I : A single group of nodes involved
      Stage-II : A single extralymphatic organ
      Stage-II : Two or more lymph node on same side of diaphragm
      Stage-III : Lymph node sites involved on both sides and diaphragm
      Stage-IV : Extralymphatic involvement.

      Investigations include blood count, LFT, X-ray chest, CT scan, bone marrow biopsy, bone scan liver biopsy, MRI scanning and staging laparotomy.

      a. Hodgkin's disease

         Survival related to stage and histological grade of tumor

         Stage-I : Involvement of single lymph node region or involvement of single extralymphatic organ or site

         Stage-II : Two or more lymph node regions involved on the same side of the diaphragm or one or more lymph node regions involved and localized involvement of extralymphatic organ on the same side of the diaphragm.

         Stage-III : Involvement of lymph node regions on both sides of the diaphragm

         Stage-IV : Disseminated involvement of one or more extralymphatic sites with or without associated lymph node involvement
         - No systemic symptoms–more favorable prognosis
         - Systemic symptoms–less favorable prognosis: Fever, sweating, weight loss and pruritis

         Histological grade : Lymphocytic predominance–favorable prognosis
         Nodular sclerosis–favorable prognosis
         Mixed cellularity–intermediate
         Lymphocytic depletion–ominous prognosis

Cytology : Eosinophils
Lymphocytes
Histiocytes
Reed-Sternberg cells
Areas of fibrosis

Spread : By involvement of adjacent lymph nodes or tissues rather than multicentric organ.

b. Investigations
- Adequate surgical biopsy
- Full blood count : Features of marrow infiltration
  - Normochromic, normocytic anaemia

  Features of hypersplenism
  - Haemolytic anaemia (with reticulocytosis)
  - Leucopenia
  - Thrombocytopenia
- Liver function tests to include serum alkaline phosphatase
- Chest X-ray : Node enlargement, especially superior mediastinum lung parenchyma involvement. Enlarged cardiac silhouette–pericardial involvement
- Skeletal survey : Deposits preferentially in ribs, spine, pelvis and bone scan
- Lymphangiography : Abnormal features
  - Enlarged nodes
  - Abnormal nodal reticular pattern
  - Filling defects in nodes
  - Abnormal sequence of opacification (shunting around lymphatic obstruction)
- Myelography : To detect extradural deposits (if indicated)
- Laparotomy : Splenectomy
  - Liver biopsy
  - Node biopsy
  - Assessment of gut involvement

c. Indication for splenectomy
- Accurate staging
  50% patients with Hodgkin's disease have splenic involvement
- Protection against marrow depression effects of radiotherapy and chemotherapy
- Prevention or treatment of hypersplenism
- Prevention of radiation damage to left kidney and left lung.

d. Treatment

Radiotherapy

- Supradiaphragmatic Stage-I: 'Mantle' irradiation
  - Cervical nodes
  - Axillary nodes
  - Mediastinal nodes
  - Normal structures shielded
- Supradiaphragmatic Stage-II: 'Mantle' irradiation + para-aortic nodes
- Intradiaphragmatic nodal disease: Inverted-'Y' field irradiation
  - Para-aortic nodes
  - Pelvic nodes
  - Inguinal nodes
  - ± Splenic axis irradiation
- Stage-IIIA: Total nodal irradiation. 'Mantle' + Inverted-'Y'

Chemotherapy

- Quadruple chemotherapy
  - Mustine
  - Vinblastine
  - Procarbazine
  - Prednisone (rapid relief systemic symptoms).

Treatment cycles of six weeks, two weeks of chemotherapy followed by an interval of four weeks to allow recovery of marrow and gastrointestinal epithelium. Treatment is continued for three four cycles after clinical remission. There is no evidence that further maintenance chemotherapy is beneficial

- Indications:
  - Stage-IV
  - Stage-IIIB
  - Adjuvant in Stage-II or IIIA to provide rapid relief of pressure on vital structures, e.g. superior vena cava.

4. Management of lymphomas is by radiotherapy Stages I and IIA and combination chemotherapy. Stages III and IV (field, Mantle or inverted). Non-Hodgkin's lymphomas are treated on similar lines except chemotherapy is introduced at earlier stage.
5. Cystic hygroma is congenital lesion made of lymph filled spaces arise from embryonic remnant of jugular lymph sac and is cavernous lymphangioma and treatment is excision.
6. Lymphoedema of unknown etiology occurring before age 35 years, lymphoedema praecox due to congenitally small lymphatics and manifest is second or third decade of life. Lymphoedema at birth is Milroy's disease. Lymphoedema occurring after age 35 is lymphoedema tarda and is because of obliteration of lymphatics.

7. Secondary lymphoedema occurs following destruction of major lymph tarda by surgery, trauma, cancer, infection or radiation most commonly involves groin to leg or axillary to arm.
8. Long standing acquired lymphoedema may predispose to lymphosarcoma. Treatment is primarily elevating graded elastic support and prevent cellulitis and lymphangitis. Reduction surgery and lymph channels are anastomosed to normal veins.
9. Carcinoma of maxillary antrum occurs in elderly, invades surrounding structures is fixed to bone. Diagnosis is by CT scan and MRI. Combination therapy with radiotherapy and surgery is used.
10. Malignant disease of tonsil is either squamous or lymphosarcoma, over 60 present with pain in throat, dysphagia and thickening of speech, ipsilateral cervical nodes are enlarged. Treatment is radiotherapy squamous cell is occasionally treated with surgical resection with radiotherapy.

CONDITIONS OF TONGUE AND CHEEK

A. Chronic superficial glossitis is characterized by leukoplakia, premalignant, atypical cells, nucleated cells and smoking, spirits spices, syphilis, sharp tooth and sepsis are etiological factors. Treatment is excision.

B. Ulceration of tongue may be:
   1. Traumatic caused by sharp tooth or denture.
   2. Aphthous ulcers are present in women, and in young men it is painful, small white ulcer. Treatment is by oral salicylate gel and topical hydrocortisone.
   3. Tuberculosis ulcer has undermined edge, treated by anti-tubercular warts and gumma of tertiary syphilis (treated by penicillin). Syphilis ulcer with snail tract ulcer, teeth, and gumma of tertiary syphilis.
   4. Carcinoma of tongue is keratinizing squamous cell carcinoma. Patient is between 60–70 years presents with pain in tongue, excessive salivation, fetor, defective speech. Posterior involves 25% bilateral to tonsillar nodes, lateral is 25% each and drains to submandibular. Central is 12.5% and tip drains to submental lymph nodes. Treatment is excision or radiotherapy. Radiotherapy is external irradiation or radioactive implants. Surgery is partial glossectomy/ hemiglossectomy with neck dissection in continuity with internal jugular vein and sternomastoid muscle. Complete resection (Commando) is extensive dissection of neck, mouth and pharynx including segment of body or ramus of mandible.

C. Oral tongue (Anterior/2/3) cancer
   1. Incidence: 36% of total cancer of oral cavity
   2. Carcinoma of tongue may present as:
      a. Oval raised and papillated plaque
      b. Ulcer

   c. Deep infected fissure
   d. Localized indurated mass.
3. Advanced cases may present as:
   a. Pain in tongue/or ear
   b. Salivation
   c. Ankyloglossia
   d. Dysphagia
   e. Improper articulation
   f. Fetor
   g. Lump in the neck.
4. *Tongue:* Squamous cell carcinoma of anterior 2/3 tongue have a predilection for lymphatic drainage to digastric, submaxillary and jugular nodes spread to submental, lower jugular is uncommon. Probability of nodal metastasis point.
   T_1 : 15% T_2 : 30% T_3 : 50% and T_4 : 75%
5. Stage-I/II: Equally effective with radiation to surgery. Curative radiation dose 6000–6500 rads by external beams 4–7 weeks. Interstitial implantation of radioactive seeds are equally effective. Surgical management requires 1–2 cm margin excision around tumor. The neck node metastasis require complete neck dissection.
6. Stage-III/IV: Treatment by wide excision of primary tumor + therapeutics neck dissection. In more advance cases post-operation radiation therapy is needed. The surgical reconstruction is based on extent of wound T_1 – primary closure or if may require clock flags, distant flap or free flaps. The overall 5 years survival rate is between 30 and 40%.

QUESTIONS AND ANSWERS

1. **What is commonest cause of enlargement of submandibular gland?**
   Ans: Generalized enlargement of submandibular gland is secondary to stone formation.
2. **What are the commonest congenital anomalies?**
   Ans: Club foot followed by cleft lip are the commonest congenital anomalies.
3. **What is optimum time for repair?**
   Ans: Cleft palate is repaired at 12–18 months before child starts to speak.
4. **What are aetiological factors for oral cancer?**
   Ans: Syphilis, sepsis, sharp tooth, spices, smoking.
5. **What is countryman lip?**
   Ans: Carcinoma of lip is called countryman lip is squamous cells carcinoma and 93% occur in lower lip.
6. **What is a thyroglossal duct cyst?**
   Ans: A thyroglossal duct cyst is a formation caused by failure of normal obliteration of the migration tract (from the foramen caecum to the normal location in the neck) of the thyroid gland.

7. **How is a parotid tumor diagnosed?**
Ans: A well-defined mass in the parotid gland as determined by physical examination is a parotid tumor until proved otherwise. Mumps, suppurative parotitis, stone in the parotid duct, and bilateral diffuse parotid enlargement would be excluded.
8. **What is the most common location of a parotid tumor?**
Ans: In the superficial lobe just beneath the lobe of the ear.
9. **What is the ratio of malignant to benign tumors of the parotid?**
Ans: At least 60% of tumors of the parotid are malignant.
10. **What is Frey's syndrome?**
Ans: Also called "gustatory sweating," this phenomenon occurs with eating in some 30% or more of patients who have had parotidectomy. It is thought to arise from regeneration of parasympathetic fibers within the auriculotemporal nerve, resulting in stimulation of the sweat glands when the parotid gland has been removed.
11. **Name the types of benign tumours of the parotid.**
Ans: Mixed tumor (the term "benign mixed tumor" has been dropped, since these lesions do recur locally and can be considered as local types of cancer). Warthin's tumors, oxyphilic adenoma, oncocystoma, and benign lymphoepithelial lesion.
12. **How is an enlarged peripheral lymph node managed?**
Soft, nontender lymph nodes of 0.5–1.0 cm are commonly palpable in the submandibular, cervical, axillary, and inguinal areas in normal individuals, and are related to infections in the mouth, pharynx, or extremities. Firm, spherical somewhat tender enlargement of a peripheral lymph node may be managed by observation over a 4 to 6 week period, some times with antibiotic therapy. However, if the enlargement does not to diagnose lymphoma or carcinoma of the oropharynx or thyroid, melanoma, or other associated malignancies. An initial needle or aspiration biopsy may be advisable.
Ans: The largest, most central node in a group is most likely to be diagnostic. Inguinal nodes often show change of chronic infection and should be avoided if other enlarged nodes are available. Biopsied nodes should be handled gently, and imprints of freshly cut surfaces should be made immediately or the node placed in a saline-soaked gauze until the pathologist can make imprints. Proper diagnosis may depend on the availability of an experienced hematopathologist.
13. **What is common cause swelling in front of tragus?**
Ans: Enlarged parotid lymph node
14. **What nerve graft is used?**
Ans: Branch of entire nerve is involved, resection would be done
15. **What is cure rate of cancer of parotid?**
Ans: Cure rate is 80–90%
16. **What are the histopathologic subtypes of malignant lymphomas?**
Ans: Hodgkin's disease is classified as nodular sclerosis (55% of cases), mixed cellularity (30%), lymphocyte predominant (10%), or lymphocyte depleted (5%). The presence of Reed-Sternberg cells is essential for the diagnosis of Hodgkin's disease. These subtypes are important for prognostic purpose, with lymphocyte predominant having the best prognosis and lymphocyte depleted the worst.
Non-Hodgkin's lymphomas have been classified in a variety of ways over the past three decades, but there has been general agreement on a "working formation" consisting of three broad, clinically relevant categories: namely, low grade, intermediate grade, and

high grade based on the predominant cell types. Within each category there are nodular lymphomas (generally have a better prognosis) and diffuse lymphomas (tend to be more aggressive), referring to the microscopic architecture of the biopsied node.

17. What is the staging system for malignant lymphoma?

The Ann Arbor classification is:

Stage-I : Involvement of a single lymph node region (I) or a single extralymphatic organ or site (IE)

Stage-II : Involvement of two or more lymph node regions on the same side of the diaphragm

Stage-III : Involvement of lymph node regions on both sides of the diaphragm. Splenic involvement plus supradiaphragmatic nodal involvement.

Stage-IV : Involvement of one or more extralymphatic organs, such as liver or bone marrow, with or without associated lymph node involvement.

Additional designations which should be added to these staging classification for prognostic and treatment-planning purpose are:

A = asymptomatic B = fever, sweats, or > 10% weight loss

18. What staging work-up should be undertaken after a malignant lymphoma has been diagnosed?

1. Detailed history and physical examination
2. Appropriate laboratory procedures
   a. Complete blood counts and erythrocyte sedimentation rate
   b. Evaluation of hepatic and renal function
3. Radiologic studies
   a. Chest roentgenogram
   b. CT scan of abdomen, pelvis, and chest
4. Lower-extremity lymphogram may occasionally indicate normal-sized with abnormal filling patterns suggestive lymphoma, and these findings may subsequent laparotomy in Hodgkin's disease. However, the presence of large retroperitoneal nodes, as in non-Hodgkin's lymphoma, may lead of life-threatening pulmonary embolization of the contrast medium. Therefore, lymphography should not be considered a routine staging procedure.
5. Skeletal roentgenograms
6. Bone marrow biopsy (if negative, repeat on opposite side)
7. The role of staging laparotomy is complex. In general, the procedure should be performed only if the result will affect therapeutic decisions. For example, if chemotherapy will be used regardless of the findings on laparotomy, there is no need for laparotomy. Hodgkin's disease that appears to be localized may be curable by radiation therapy if all involved nodes are included in the treatment field, therapy justifying laparotomy and biopsy of retroperitoneal nodes. Non-Hodgkin's lymphomas are usually treated with chemotherapy because of widespread nodal and extranodal involvement (especially of the bone marrow). And therefore, laparotomy is often considered not to be necessary for treatment planning.

19. How are malignant lymphomas treated?

Ans: Stage IA and IIA Hodgkin disease has cure rate 90% after radiation therapy such as extended mantle field of total nodal irradiation. Stage IIB, III, IV are treated with adriamycin + bleomycin + vinblastine + dacarbazine (ABVD) alternating with nitrogen mustard + vincristine + procarbazine + prednisone (MOPP). Long-term complete remission are expected in 70–90% of patients treated with this regimen. Unfavorable histology (mixed cellularity of lymphocyte depleted) usually calls for the use of chemotherapy, with or without radiation therapy, even when the disease seems to be localized, because of the relapse rates seen after use of radiation therapy alone.

Non-Hodgkin's lymphomas are generally treated with systemic combination chemotherapy, such as cyclophosphamide, adriamycin oncovin, and prednisone (CHOP), because they are often generalized when the first present. Even more intensive regimens intermediate-grade or high-grade lymphomas), because about half of patients will respond to intensive chemotherapy with long-term remission, and presumably many patients are cured.

20. **Contrast the incidence curves for Hodgkin's disease and the non-Hodgkin's lymphomas?**
Ans: For Hodgkin's disease, there is a bimodal incidence with one peak in the 20s and a second in the 60s. Non-Hodgkin's lymphomas rise steadily in incidence from childhood through 80 years of age.

21. **What are the staging tests used for Hodgkin's disease?**
Ans: Any non-nodal involvement other than the spleen indicates stage IV disease. Therefore, one of the first tests used is bilateral bone marrow biopsies. If positive, one need only pursue work-up of other potential problem areas such as renal obstruction. A chest X-ray is mandatory. Lymphangiography in good hands is about 85% accurate in diagnosing periaortic nodes below the renal arteries; however, CT scanning is more sensitive for upper abdominal nodes. A chest CT scan frequently detects otherwise occult mediastinal disease. If liver function tests are abnormal, a liver biopsy may be required.

22. **What are the pathologic subtypes of Hodgkin's disease?**
Ans: There are (in rough order of frequency) nodular sclerosis (35%), mixed cellularity (33%). Lymphocyte-predominant (16%), and lymphocyte-depleted (16%), nodular sclerosis does very well in stage I or II when treated by radiation therapy alone but has the second-highest relapse rate when stage III or IV disease is treated with chemotherapy.

Flow Chart: Hodgkin's disease

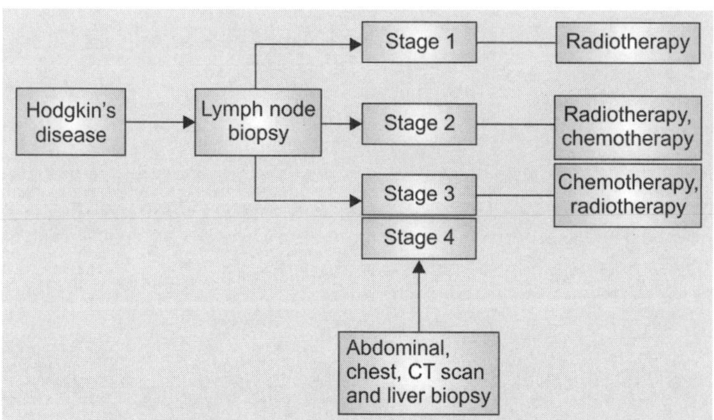

Flow Chart: Neck mass

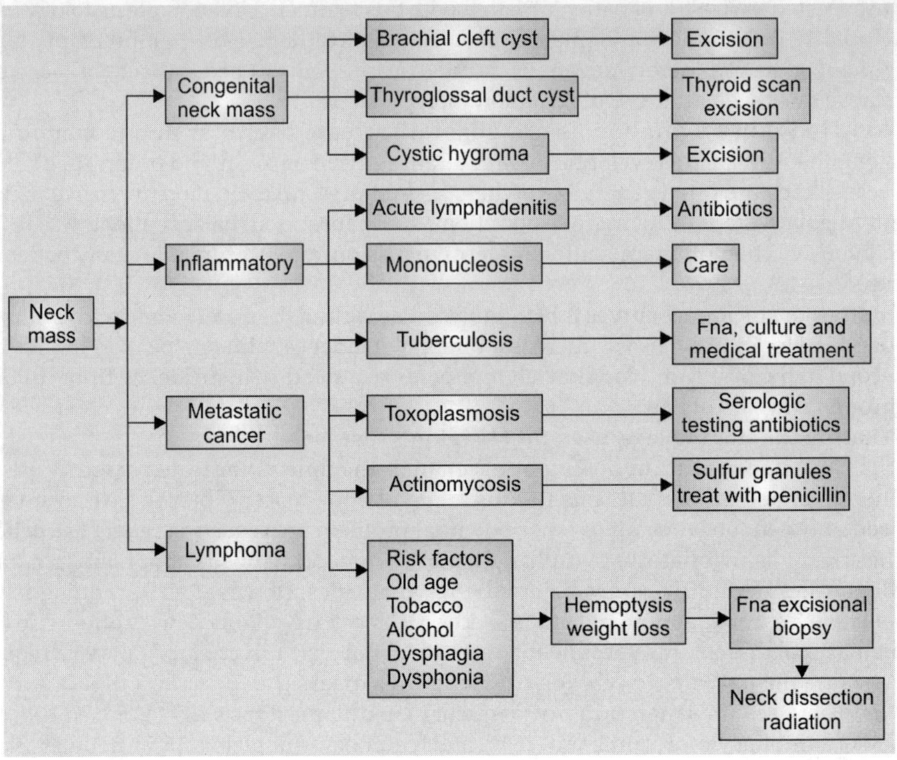

6 Change of Bowel Habits and Bleeding

Change of bowel habits is usually insidious and may be increasing constipation or alternate periods of diarrhoea and constipation. Bleeding could be due to bleeding disorders or inherent abdominal cause.

UPPER BLEEDING

The most common cause is peptic ulcer disease. The other cause are gastritis in alcoholics non-alcoholics and esophageal varices.

Treatment should include IV hydration, endoscopy, sclerotherapy, esophageal balloons and definite surgical operations. In children most common causes is esophageal varices.

LOWER BLEEDING

Resuscitative efforts and coagulation defect corrections.

Hematochezia is more than 1 liter of blood loss per rectum and arteriography helps in diagnosis (3–4 ml/min).

Tagged RBCs studies help to locate bleeding for amounts less than 2 ml/min. Gastrointestinal losses may lead to melaena.

The most common cause of massive GI bleeding is diverticulosis of colon. Telangiectasis (AV malformation of colonic wall, ulcerative colitis, carcinoma colon, colonic and rectal polyp are other causes of lower GI bleeding.

Instusseption and polyps are most common causes of lower GI bleeding in children.

After diagnosis, endoscopic definitive surgical treatment is required.

QUESTIONS AND ANSWERS

1. **What is upper gastrointestinal (UGI) bleeding?**
   Ans: UGI bleeding occurs from lesions of the GI tract located form the oropharynx to the ligament of Treitz. The usual presentation is that of Hematemesis and melaena.
2. **What are the five most frequent causes of UGI bleeding, their relative frequency, and the success of medical management?**
   a. Gastritis is the most frequent cause of UGI bleeding–approximately 40% of patients; success of medical management in controlling bleeding is 90%.
   b. Duodenal ulcers are the source of bleeding in 7% of patients; medical management is successful in 75%.

c. Gastric ulcers are the source in 15% of patients; medical management is successful in only 60%.
d. Mallory-Weiss tears are found in 11% of patients; medical management is 95% successful.
e. Esophagogastric varices occur in 8%; medical management is successful in only 50%.

Ans: Other less frequent causes are gastric neoplasms (carcinoma, leiomyomas, leiomyosarcomas, and lymphomas), hiatal or paraesophageal hernias, haemobilia, arteriovenous malformations, angiodysplasias, duodenal diverticular, visceral artery aneurysms, aortoduodenal fistulas, and polyps.

3. **What is the natural history of UGI hemorrhage?**
Ans: 85% of patients hospitalized with UGI hemorrhage will stop bleeding with routine medical management; 15% will require emergent operative intervention.
4. **Which salient features of a patient's history must be obtained?**
a. Presentation of bleeding (Hematemesis–UGI, hematochezia–UGI or LGI, bleeding melena probably UGI and occult blood.
b. Duration of bleeding; presence of orthostatic symptoms.
c. Significant past history, especially prior symptoms or diagnosis of peptic ulcer disease or prior GI bleed. Also inquire about prior surgery and significant medical history, including cardiac, pulmonary, vascular, or hepatic problems. Any patient with cirrhosis should be evaluated carefully and child's classification (A,B,C,) determined.
d. Precipitating factors (history of retching or vomiting history of drug abuse, including alcohol, ethyalcohol, salicylates, steroids, NSAIDs and smoking.
e. Age (patients over 60 years tolerate a large UGI bleed poorly).
5. **How much blood loss is necessary to cause melena?**
Ans: As little as 50 cc of blood can cause clinically obvious melena. With a bleed of 1000 cc, melena can persists for 5 days and stool can remain Hemoccult-positive for 3 weeks.
6. **What is haemobilia? What are the symptoms?**
Ans: Haemobilia is a rare disorder described as an abnormal connection between hepatic blood vessels and bile ducts. Trauma is the most frequent cause. Symptoms include intermittent, colicky right upper quadrant pain, jaundice and Hematemesis.
7. **What is the most common cause of UGI bleeding in children?**
Ans: Portal hypertension secondary to extrahepatic portal vein obstruction with bleeding esophageal and gastric varices is the most common cause of massive, bleeding and foreign bodies in children, and swallowed maternal blood in neonates.
8. **What initial steps should be taken in the work-up and management of a patient with significant UGI bleeding?**
a. Rapid assessment and resuscitation of hemorrhagic shock, including large-bore lines and fluid replacement.
b. History and physical exam
c. Nasogastric (NG) to confirm diagnosis, to clear the stomach of blood, and to assess continued bleeding.
d. Hematocrit may be unreliable initially equilibration taken 4–8 hours, but should be monitored every 4–6 hours, (b) PT/PTT and platelet count to rule out coagulopathy, and (c) liver function tests to rule out underlying liver disease.
e. Type and cross-match blood.

f. Consider early esophagogastroduodenoscopy (EGD) to confirm diagnosis and source of hemorrhage and to assess amount of active bleeding.
g. Foley catheter to monitor urine output.
h. Early surgical consultation.

9. What are the best methods for diagnosis acute UGI hemorrhage?

a. NG, false negative 1% must have bilious returns to be certain one is not missing a duodenal source. False positive 7% secondary to NG trauma.
b. Upper gastrointestinal endoscopy is the most reliable method (90–95%) accuracy and is the gold standard.
c. Selective angiography of the celiac axis and superior mesenteric artery is 90% accurate if blood loss is at least 4–5 cc/min, and is 20% accurate for varices in venous phase film. In general, however, angiography has more value in diagnosing lower GI hemorrhage and is used infrequently in patients with UGI bleeding.
d. Upper GI contrast series are rarely useful and have low yield in the setting of acute UGI bleeding (56% accurate for ulcers, 50% accurate for varices, 24% false-negative rate).
e. Laparotomy for emergent situations in which other studies have been inconclusive.

10. What endoscopic methods are available to control UGI bleeding?

Ans: Endoscopic sclerotherapy is successful in acutely controlling variceal hemorrhage in over 90% of cases, with a mortality of less than 10%. Whether repeated sclerotherapy affects long-term prognosis in patients with esophageal varices is yet to be determined. Operative intervention carries a 50–75% mortality.

Endoscopic techniques for nonvariceal hemorrhage include a variety of thermal coagulation and injection techniques. The thermal methods include laser photocoagulation (YAG or argon), monopolar or bipolar electrocoagulation, and direct application of heat using "heater probe". Injection therapy methods involve injection of substances, either vasoconstrictors such as epinephrine or sclerosing agents such as 98% ethanol and polidocan. Moreover, less expensive and simple methods of hemostasis (e.g., heater probe and injection therapy) appear to be as effective as the laser.

11. What are indications of operative interventional?

a. Persistent shock with active bleeding.
b. Blood loss of 2500 cc during the first 24 hours or 1500 cc during the second 24 hours.
c. Recurrent bleeding during the initial hospitalization while on maximal medical therapy.
d. Significant history of or recurrent bleeding from peptic ulcer disease.
e. Association illness or advanced age, which makes patients poor risks for tolerating recurrent hemorrhage.

12. What are the surgical options for treatment of the five most common causes of UGI bleeding?

a. *Gastritis:* Vagotomy and pyloroplasty or Vagotomy and antrectomy. Total gastrectomy generally not advocated as an initial procedure because of the prohibitive mortality (100%) in critically ill patients.
b. *Duodenal ulcer:* ligation of the bleeding vessel and Vagotomy and pyloroplasty, Vagotomy and antrectomy, highly selective Vagotomy.
c. *Gastric ulcer:* Vagotomy and pyloroplasty or hemigastrectomy with or without Vagotomy. All ulcers must be biopsied to rule out malignant disease, and preferably wedged but if not included in a standard gastric resection.

d. *Mallory-Weiss tears:* oversewing of tears
e. *Esophagogastric varices:* Emergent (Child's A or B portocaval or mesocaval shunt nonselective portal decompression). Emergent (Child's C): do not operate portocaval or mesocanal shunt, esophageal devscularization (modified Sugiura procedure. Semielective Child's A or B): strongly consider a distal splenorenal shunt (selective decompression).

13. **Is diverticulitis the most common cause of massive lower GI bleeding in adults?**
Ans: No. Diverticulitis or inflammation of colonic diverticulosis rarely presents with blood loss. Diverticulosis, seen in >60% of patients over the age of 60, is the most common cause of massive hemorrhage from the lower GI tract. Of all patients with diverticulosis, only a small minority (5%) will have a major bleeding episode.

14. **Can bleeding from the stomach or duodenum present with the passage of bright red blood rectally?**
Ans: Yes. The color of passed blood is a function of gastrointestinal transit time. A briskly bleeding lesion of the stomach or duodenum with subsequent quick passage of blood though the GI tract can present with bright red blood per rectum and often hypotension of shock. Melena (the passage of black, tarry stools) is caused by the chemical interaction of gastric acid with blood over several hours to form hematin.

15. **What are the nonhaemorrhagic causes of dark stools?**
Ans: Inquiries as to the ingestion of iron, lico, or bismuth-containing compounds must be made at the initial evaluation of a patient who present with dark from ingestion of such compounds lack the "tarry" character of melena.

16. **Who two radionuclide tests are currently available for identifying bleeding in the GI tract?**
Ans: The 99 m-technetium (Tc) sulfur colloid scan and the 99 m-Tc red cell scan are currently available and have different potential benefits. The sulfur colloid scan is similar to arteriography in that it must be used in the actively bleeding patient for the study to be positive. Its advocates claim that test can detect bleeding rates as low as 0.1 ml/min. A major disadvantage lies with test inability to provide accurate information on the origin of bleeding detected in delayed scans.

17. **What is the most common site of bleeding colonic diverticular?**
Ans: While colonic diverticula are most prevalent in the left side of the colon, bleeding diverticular occur more often on the right side.

18. **What rate of blood loss into the bowel is necessary for accurate localization of bleeding by arteriography?**
Ans: A rate of blood loss of at least 1.5–2 cc/min is necessary for angiography to be useful.

19. **Where are arteriovenous malformations of the colon located?**
Ans: The caecum is the most common location, but they have been found in the ileum, ascending colon, and hepatic flexure. When present, there are usually several.

20. **What are the generally accepted indications for operative intervention in the management of lower GI bleeding?**
Ans: Patients requiring more than 5 units of whole blood within the first 6 hours despite aggressive medical or angiographic management should undergo exploratory surgery. Surgery should be performed in any patient who rebleeds after initial stabilization with conservative therapy.

21. **What is the proper surgical treatment of a patient with known diverticulosis, chronic intermittent rectal bleeding, and arteriovenous malformation?**
Ans: Both right hemicolectomy and subtotal colectomy have been advocated. There is growing evidence, however, that right hemicolectomy alone may be adequate.

22. **What is Rendu-Osler-Weber disease?**
Ans: Also known as hereditary hemorrhagic telangiectasia, this syndrome is transmitted as an autosomal dominant trait and is characterized by increased fragility of the small arteries and veins of the mucous membranes of the nasopharynx and GI tract, resulting in bleeding. Pulmonary arteriovenous malformations and hepatic cirrhosis are other feature of this disease.

23. **What is cause of the massive bleeding in pediatric group?**
Ans: Meckel's diverticulum

24. **How much blood loss is required for stool guaiac test?**
Ans: 10 ml/day

Flow Chart: Upper GI bleeding

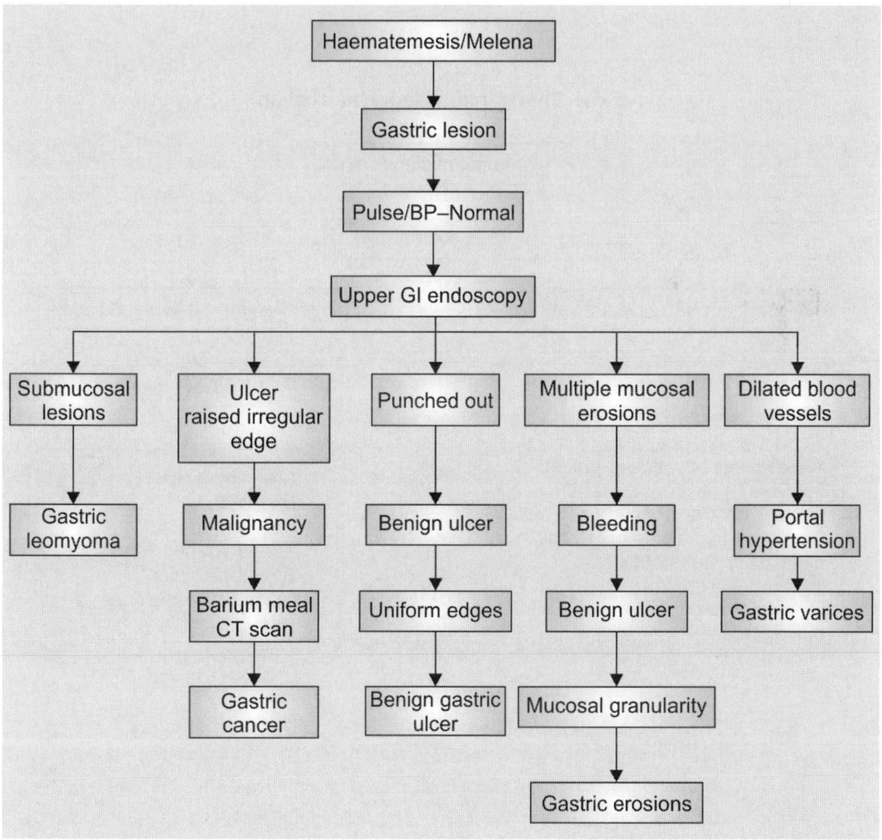

Flow Chart: Lower gastrointestinal bleeding

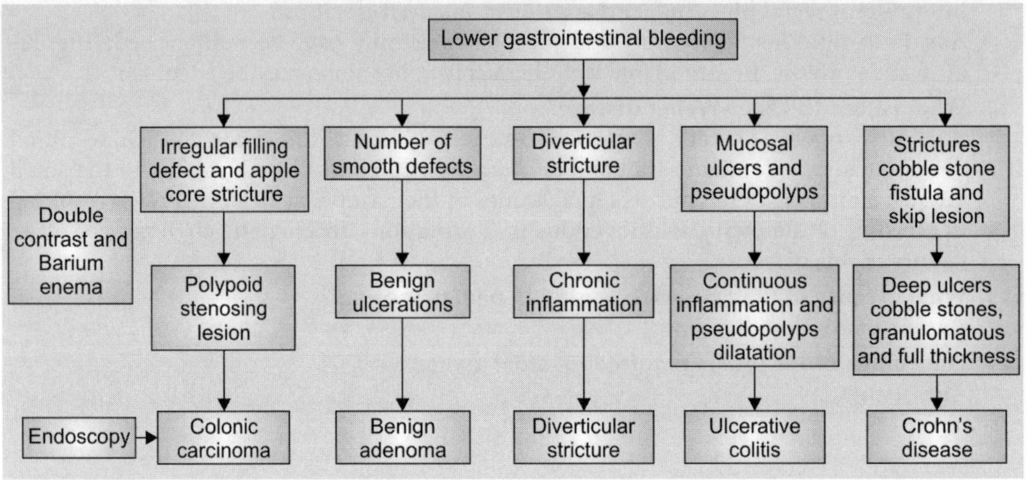

Flow Chart: Intermittent claudication

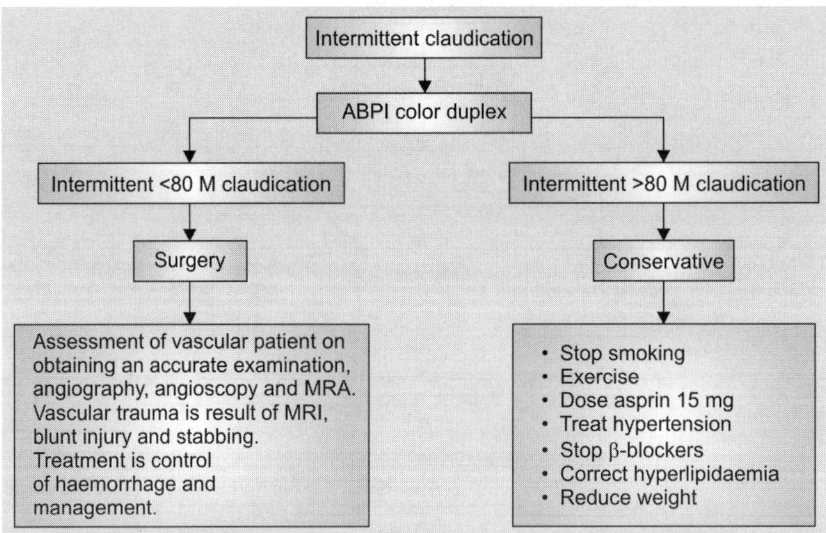

Flow Chart: Lower GI bleeding

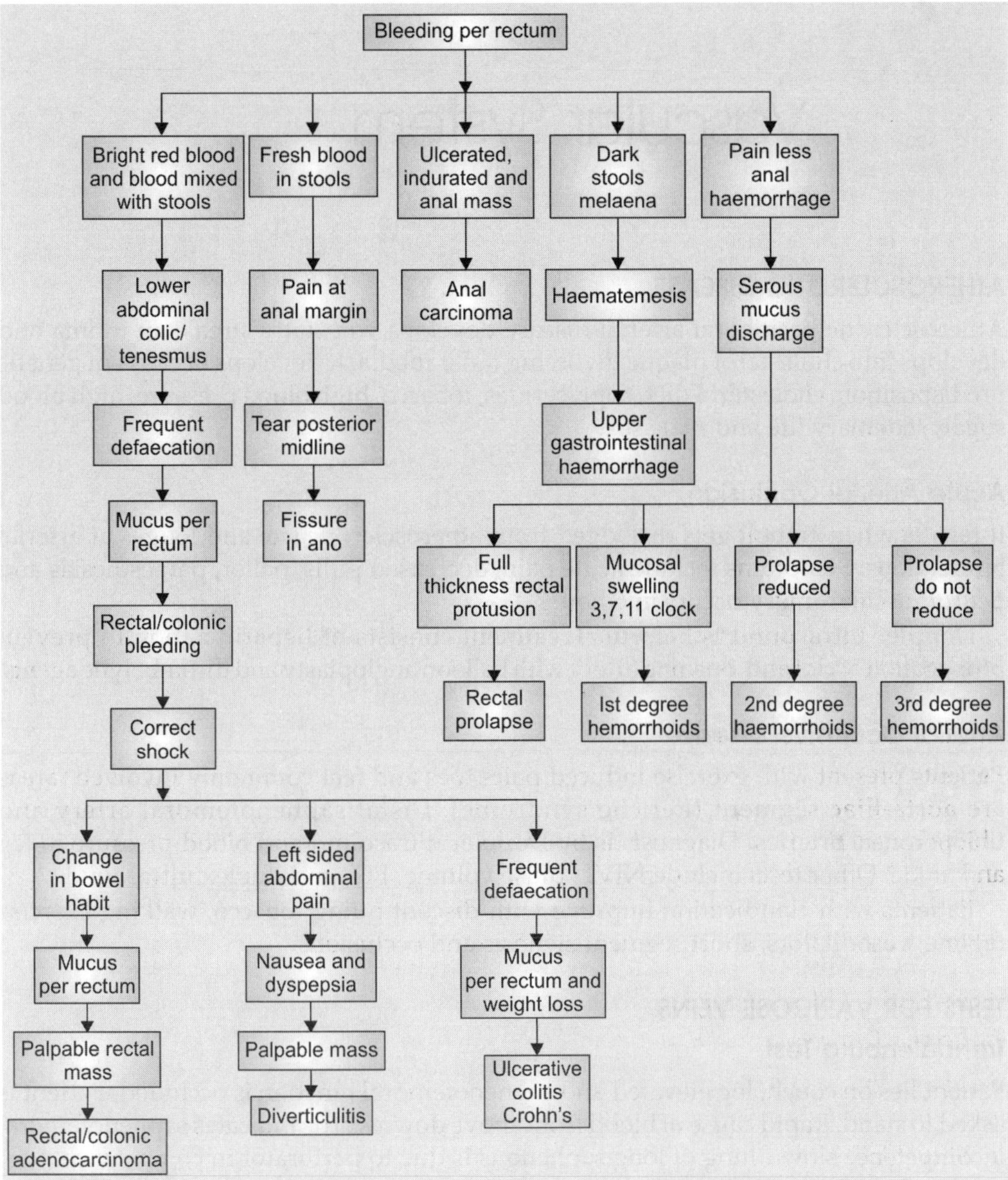

7

Vascular System

ATHEROSCLEROTIC DISEASE

Atherosclerotic peripheral arterial disease develops with fatty streaks in intima and develops into cholesterol plaque involving inner media. It develops because of genetic predisposition, cholesterol diet, triglycerides, tobacco, high blood pressure, high blood sugar, sedentary life and male sex.

Acute Arterial Occlusion

It results when emboli gets dislodged from atherosclerotic site and lodges at arterial bifurcations. Symptoms include acute pain, decreased pulls, pallor, paraesthesias and neuromuscular injury occurs in 6 hours.

Doppler ultrasound is helpful. Treatment consists of heparinization to prevent propagation of clot and opening artery with balloon angioplasty and thrombolytic agents.

Arterial Occlusive Disease

Patients present with exercise induced pairs toes and feet commonly involved areas are aorta-iliac segment (Leriche syndrome). Distal saphenofemoral artery and tibioperoneal arteries. Diagnosis is by Doppler ultrasound and blood pressure in leg and ankle. Other tests include NIVL, pulse volume, PO_2 and duplex ultrasound.

Patients with claudication improve with discontinuing tobacco, walking exercise regime, vasodilators, short segment stenosis and occlusions.

TESTS FOR VARICOSE VEINS

Trendelenburg Test

Patient lies on couch, leg elevated and saphenofemoral junction is occluded. Patient is asked to stand. Rapid cause of blood from above downwards indicates saphenofemoral incompetence slow filling of long saphenous is due to perforator in competence.

Multiple Tourniquet

Four tourniquet are applied at various levels.

1st tourniquet	:	At level of saphenofemoral junction
2nd tourniquet	:	At level of middle of thigh to occlude perforator in hunter canal
3rd tourniquet	:	Below knee
4th tourniquet	:	Lower-third of leg above medial malleolus.

Appearance of veins between 1st and 2nd indicates in competence of thigh perforators, 2nd and 3rd indicates incompetence of knee perforators, 3rd and 4th indicates incompetence of ankle perforators.

Causes of deep vein thrombosis

Trauma–injury to vessel
Increased coagulability
Road traffic accidents
Operations
Malignancy
Blood disorders polycythaemia
Orthopaedic surgery
Serious illness
Immobilization

Maximum incidence on 2nd day. Postoperative period with dilated veins, dull aching pain and low grade fever.

Phlegmasia alba dolens occurs when thrombus extends calf region to iliofemoral vein.

Phlegmasia coerulea dolens refers to blue leg with loss of superficial tissues of toes.

1. Diagnostic evaluation includes Duplex U/S to assess the degree of stenosis and the morphology of the plaque and/or OPG (oculopneumoplethysmography) to indirectly gauge the degree of stenosis. CT scan or MR scan often reveal previous undetected cerebral scans.
2. Arteriography is usually done prior to operation to look for AS disease in sites other than the carotid bifurcation (aortic arch, intracranial, etc.).
3. Risk of stroke in a patient with TIAs is 5–6% year and two recent studies have shown superior patient outcome when symptomatic patients with >75% stenosis are treated with carotid endarterectomy. Expected perioperative stroke rate 2–4%, mortality 1–2%.
4. Asymptomatic patient with critical stenoses (>90%) may do better with endarterectomy versus ASA alone if perioperative stroke rate is <2%.
5. Recurrent symptomatic rate after CEA is approximately 1%/year (similar to population) but restenosis rate may be 10–15%.
6. Bilateral carotid disease along with bilateral vertebral artery disease may lead to "vertebrobasilar symptoms" of paraplegia, dizziness plus speech or hemiplegia problems, bilateral blindness episodes, etc. may be improved by carotid endarterectomy (or occasionally repair/revision of vertebral artery).
7. Subclavian steal syndrome is the onset of vertebrobasilar symptoms with exercise of left arm, due to occlusion of left subclavian artery proximal to vertebral artery, resulting in reversal of flow in the vertebral to supply the arm. Symptoms improve with carotid-subclavian bypass of PTA of subclavian artery. If patient has no symptoms, nothing is done.

Non-artherosclerotic Arterial Disease

1. Raynaud's syndrome–a vasospastic disorder, more common in women than men, of unknown etiology, manifested by abnormally severe reaction of fingers and

hands to cold exposure. Usually a benign condition treated with gloves or low-dose vasodilating agents, i.e. calcium channel blockers. May be associated with other autoimmune disorders, i.e. SLE, anticardiolipin antibody syndrome, scleroderma, rheumatoid arthritis, etc.

2. Buerger's disease–arteritis obliterans–a disease of smokers, men > women, involving progressive obliteration of small and medium sized arteries of the hands and feet. Commonly leads to amputations. Treatment involves complete abstinence from tobacco.
3. Polyarteritis nodosa–autoimmune complex disease that can lead to microaneurysm formation or obliterative processes in the small vessels.
4. Deep venous system comprises of femoral popliteal veins, renal comitantes, anterior tibial posterotibial, peroneal arteries and veins draining calf muscles. High pressure system supported by powerful muscles.

Venous Disease

A. Deep Vein Thrombosis (DVT)

1. Etiology–Virchow's triad–stasis, vessel injury, hypercoagulable state.
2. High-risk groups for development include females, elderly, overweight, immobile, cancer, previous history of DVT, orthopedic procedures, etc.
3. Preventive measure include low dose heparin (5000 units it hourly), calf pumps, early ambulation. For orthopedic patients, dextran or full anticoagulation.
4. Diagnosis–clinical signs/symptoms of painful, swollen calf with + Homan's sign is only approximately 50 percent accurate.

Destruction of Values

Inferior vena cava–no valve
Common iliac vein–no valve
Long saphenous vein–10-1 valve
Short saphenous vein–1 valve

a. Non-invasive tests include duplex ultrasound, impedance plethysmography, and venous Doppler exam.
b. Venography is the radiographic choice.

5. Treatment is anticoagulation for 6–12 weeks, first with heparin, then with warfarin.
6. Thrombolytic agents dissolve clots faster but are more expensive and ultimate value are still in question.
7. Complications of DVT include pulmonary emboli (PE) and venous valvular insufficiency (postphlebitic syndrome).

PULMONARY EMBOLISM

1. Common cause of contributing factor to deaths in the hospital.
2. Manifestations includes sudden chest pain, SOB, tachypnea, feeling of impending doom, hypoxia occasionally hemoptysis. There are often absent.

3. Diagnosis most reliable made with pulmonary angiogram. Nuclear lung scans are used commonly and can be helpful along with chest X-ray and compatible clinical scenario.
4. Treatment usually involves 3–6 months anticoagulation (heparin followed by warfarin) but thrombolytics may have value in lysing clots faster and more thoroughly, leading to less long-term pulmonary arterial resistance.
5. Patients with recurrent PE in anticoagulation, complications to anticoagulants or contraindication to anticoagulation should be protected with an IVC filter (Greenfield or "Bird's nest" filters are most commonly used).

VENOUS VALVULAR INSUFFICIENCY

1. Causes include malformed valves, chronic stress leading to valve failure, and injury to the valve after thrombosis.
2. Superficial valvular incompetence leads to varicose veins which can be treated with graded elastic support or, if symptoms such as phlebitis, bleeding or severe cosmetic deformity result, can be excised (stripping).

Varicose Veins

A. Dilated tortuous superficial veins affecting lower limbs. They are found in distribution of long saphenous vein and less frequently of short saphenous vein and commonest abnormality incompetence at saphenofemoral symptoms include acting on prolonged standing and occasional itching.
B. Assessment in by inspection, by use of tourniquet with Trendelenburg's test to identify the level of reflux. Tapping test can be done by tapping the proximal vein in the region of saphenofemoral junction will cause a thrill detected by a hand placed distally. Hand help Doppler insonation and color duplex is an excellent tool for complex venous disease. Photoplethysmography useful for identifying patients with venous pump dysfunction.
C. Saphenofemoral incompetence requires flush saphenofemoral ligation (Trendenburg's) and strip the long saphenous from groin to knee stripping the vein below knee and superficial varicosities are dealt with multiple stab phelotrotomy. Incompetent perforatory veins in leg are treated with subfascial ligation which can be carried endoscopically.
D. Injection sclerotherapy or laser coagulation is reversed by superficial varicosities in leg in absence of saphenofemoral or saphenopopliteal incompetence stockings are worn for 4 weeks and patient is encouraged to walk daily for 4 weeks venous ulceration is significant problem and adequate compression therapy 74% of ulcer within 12 weeks. Color duplex assessment ABI >0.8 is essential.

Vascular Trauma

Majority is result of blunt injury, fracture or stabbing. Treatment is control of hemorrhage.

Surgical sympathetomy is correctly performed for hyperhidrosis of hands or axilla. The thoracoscopic sympathectomy diathermied, resects 2nd and 3rd ganglia, lumbar sympathectomy L2 and L3 ganglia it is done by open or laparoscopic approach.

Minimal invasive vascular surgery such as subfacial endoscopic perforation surgery, endoscopic saphenous vein harvesting, thoracoscopic sympathectomy and laparoscopic sympathectomy are becoming popular.

QUESTIONS AND ANSWERS

1. **What is claudication?**
   Ans: Claudication is exercise induced intermittent discomfort in a particular muscle group which promptly subsides within 1 to 5 minutes after the exercise is stopped. This discomfort may be described by the patient as pain, cramping, burning, or weariness. In the lower extremities the calf, thigh, and buttocks are most frequently affected. Because the pain is reproducible by the same amount of exertion, it is typically quantifies by the distance a patient can walk prior to onset.

2. **What is the pathophysiology of claudication?**
   Ans: The symptoms of claudication result from relative hypoxia in a particular muscle group when its increased metabolic demands for oxygen during exercise cannot be met. Although normal arteries can increase flow by 5 to 10 fold when regional metabolic demands rise, stenosed or occluded vessels have an extremely limited capacity to augment flow during exercise. The stenosis or occlusion is invariably secondary to progressive atherosclerosis.

3. **What is the differential diagnosis of lower extremity pain?**
   Ans: Claudication is a characteristic symptom of patients with significant arterial occlusive disease. Because of the reproducible characteristics of hypoxic muscle pain with exercise, a history and physical examination should be sufficient to rule out most other cases.
   1. *Acute arterial embolus:* The resultant precipitous reduction of blood flow will cause an acute onset of diffuse lower extremity pain at rest in a pain at rest in a patient with no history of arterially occlusive disease.
   2. *Chronic venous disease:* Venous valve incompetence and resultant relative stasis causes chronic swelling, hyperpigmentation, and ulcers at or proximal to the malleoli.
   3. *Deep venous thrombosis:* Deep vein thrombosis may cause extremity swelling or vague pain, history and physical examination are notoriously inaccurate in making this diagnosis.
   4. *Musculoskeletal disorder:* This is associated by a history of pain in association with movement of a joint or recent trauma.
   5. *Neurologic disorders:* Lumbar disc herniation or spinal stenosis may cause characteristic "shooting" pain or extremity weakness, which should be distinct from claudication.
   6. *Infection:* Local erythema and tenderness should be present that is not exacerbated by exercise.

4. **What are the signs of significant arterial occlusive disease?**
   Ans: Signs that may be appreciated at physical examination include: (1) absent distal pulses; (2) pallor of the extremity on elevation and rubor on its dependency; (3) trophic changes such as thinning of the skin. Loss of hair, and thickening of the nails; (4) muscle atrophy and (5) tissue loss (ulcers distal to the malleolus gangrene).

5. **What is an appropriate initial treatment for claudication?**
Ans: In keeping with the natural history of this disease, a conservative initial approach is warranted. This includes:
   i. *Smoking cessation:* Tobacco use is clearly associated with a significant exacerbation of vascular occlusive disease. Smoking doubles an elderly patient's risk of claudication. Most claudication smokers can expect significant improvement in exercise tolerance by quitting.
   ii. *Exercise:* A graded exercise program will stimulate collateral vessel formation. The resultant increase in blood flow can improve walking by 80 to 120%.
   iii. *Analysis and control of blood lipids:* Any patient with claudication should maintain his or her ideal body weight and have a lipid panel checked and controlled with an appropriate diet and , if needed, drug therapy (e.g., niacin, lovastatin).
   iv. *Pentoxifylline (Trental):* This exerts its effect by lowering blood viscosity. The mechanism underlying this action is not completely understood but may include increasing erythrocyte flexibility and decreasing platelet aggregation. These actions may provide enchanced perfusion to areas with high-grade stenoses or small collaterals. It use has been demonstrated to be beneficial in some, but not all, studies. Similar benefits can be achieved with a good exercise program. Although conflicting data concerning efficacy and its high cost make the drug's widespread use somewhat controversial, the trend is toward greater use in a selected group of patients.

6. **What is rest pain? What causes rest pain?**
Ans: Rest pain is caused by inadequate delivery of oxygen to the tissues at rest. The hypoperfusion commonly manifests itself as ischemic pain in the foot at rest.

7. **What is peripheral vascular disease (PVD)?**
Ans: Occulasive atherosclerotic disease in the lower extremities.

8. **What is the most common site of arterial atherosclerotic occlusion in the lower extremities?**
Ans: Occlusion of the SFA in Hunter's canal.

9. **What are the symptoms of PVD?**
Ans: Intermittent claudication, rest pain, erectile dysfunction, sensory motor impairment, tissue loss.

10. **What is intermittent pain?**
Ans: Pain, cramping , or both of the lower extremity, usually the calf muscle, after walking a specific distance, then the pain/cramping resolves after stopping for a specific amount of time while standing this pattern is reproducible.

11. **What is pain?**
Ans: Pain is the foot, usually over the distal metatarsals, this pain arises at rest (classically at night, awakening the patient).

12. **What are the signs of PVD?**
Ans: Absent pulses bruits, muscular atrophy, decreased hair growth, thick toenails, tissue necrosis/ulcers/infection.

13. **What is the ABI?**
Ans: The Ankle to Brachial Index (ABI) simply the ratio of systolic blood pressure at the ankle to the systolic blood pressure at the arm (brachial artery) Ankle pressure is taken with Doppler.

14. **What are the indicator for surgical treatment in PVD?**
Ans: (1) Rest pain, (2) Tissue necrosis, (3) Infection, (4) Severe claudication refractory to conservative treatment that affects quality of life/livelihood.
15. **What is the treatment of claudication?**
Ans: For the vast majority, conservative treatment, including exercise, smoking cessation, treatment of HTN, diet, aspirin, with or without Trental (pentoxifylline).
16. **How can you remember the medical conservative treatment for claudication?**
Ans: The acronym **PACE:** P Pentoxifylline, A Asprin, C Cessation of smoking, E Exercise distal aorta.
17. **What is a Femoral popliteal bypass?**
Ans: By pass SFA occlusion with a graft from the femoral artery to the popliteal artery.
18. **What is a Femorodistal bypass?**
Ans: Bypass from the femoral artery to a distal (peroneal artery, anterior tibial artery, or posterior tibial artery).
19. **What are the indications of lower extremity amputations?**
Ans: Irreversible tissue ischemia (no hope for revascularization bypass) and necrotic tissue, severe infection, severe pain with no bypassable vessels, or if patient is not interested in a bypass procedure.
20. **What is acute arterial occlusion?**
Ans: Acute occlusion of an artery, usually by embolization, other causes include acute thrombosis of an artheromatous lesion, vascular trauma.
21. **What are the classic signs/symptoms of acute arterial occlusion?**
Ans: The six Ps : pain paralysis, pallor, paresthesia, polar (poikilothermia), pulselessness.
22. **What is the most common cause of embolus from the heart?**
Ans: A-fib
23. **What is the treatment of acute arterial occlusion?**
Ans: Surgical embolectomy via cutdown and Fogarty balloon (bypass is reversed for embolectomy failure).
24. **What is acute mesenteric ischemia?**
Ans: Acute onset of intestinal ischemia.
25. **What are the causes of acute mesenteric ischemia?**
Ans: (1) Emboli to mesenteric vessel from the heart, (2) Acute thrombosis of long-standing atherosclerosis of mesenteric artery.
26. **What is the treatment of a mesenteric embolus?**
Ans: Perform Fogarty catheter embolectomy, resect obviously necrotic intestine, and leave marginal looking bowel until a second look laparotomy is performed 24 to 72 hours post-operatively.
27. **What is median arcuate ligament syndrome?**
Ans: Mesenteric ischemia resulting from narrowing of the celiac axis vessels by extrinsic compression by the median arcuate ligament.
28. **What is pulmonary embolism (PE)?**
Ans: DVT that embolizes to the pulmonary arterial system.
29. **What is DVT?**
Ans: Deep venous thrombosis–a clot forming in the pelvic or lower extremity veins.

30. Is DVT more common in the right or left iliac vein?
Ans: Left is more common (4 to 1) becomes the aortic bifurcation crosses and possibly compresses the left iliac vein.

31. What are the signs/symptoms of DVT?
Ans: Lower extremity pain, swelling, tenderness, Homan's sign, pulmonary embolus (PE). Up to 50% can be asymptomatic !

32. What is Homan's sign?
Ans: Calf pain with dorsiflexion of the foot seen classically with DVT, but actually found in fewer than one-third of patients with DVT.

33. What test is used to evaluate for DVT?
Ans: Duplex ultrasonography.

34. What is Virchow's triad?
Ans: Stasis, endothelial injury, hypercoagulable state (risk factors for thrombosis).

35. What are the risk factors for DVT and PE?
Ans: Postoperative status, multiple trauma, paralysis, immobility, CHF, obesity, BCP/ tamoxifen, cancer, advanced age, polycythemia, MI, HIT syndrome, hypercoagulable state (protein C/protein S deficiency).

36. What are the signs/symptoms?
Ans: Shortness of breath, tachypnea, hypotension, CP, occasionally fever, tender LE, loud pulmonic component of S_2, hemoptysis with pulmonary infarct.

37. What are the associated lab findings?
Ans: ABG–decreased PO_2 and PCO_2 (from hyperventilation).

38. Which diagnostic tests are indicated?
Ans: (1) Westermark's sign (wedge-shaped area of decreased pulmonary vasculature resulting in hyperlucency), (2) Opacity with base at pleural edge from pulmonary infarction.

Flow Chart: Thromboembolism

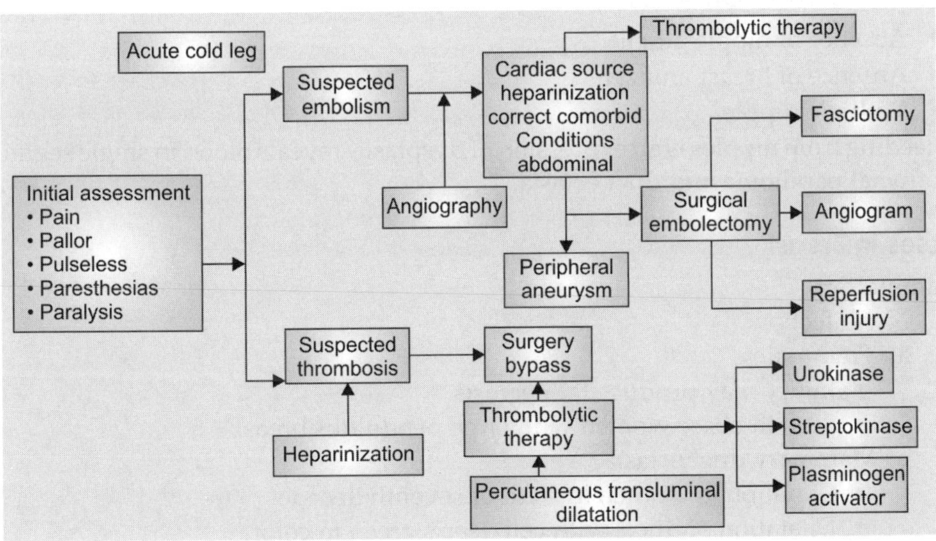

8

Breast

ANATOMY

- Extends between 2nd and 6th costal cartilages.
- On three muscular pectoral's–major, serratus anterior and external oblique but separated from these by deep fascia.
- Secretary acinic embedded into stroma grouped as lobules. Each lobe (15–20 lobules). Drained by single duct, open and forum coalescence of ducts at nipple separated by septa.
- Blood supply is lateral thoracic, perforating branches of internal mammary and lateral branches of 2nd, 3rd, 4th intercostals arteries. Veins-plexus beneath areola drain into internal mammary.
- Lymph glands receive lymph from breast. Anterior chin under pectoral muscles (pectoral nodes level 1) first to be involved in breast cancer. Posterior chain on post wall of axilla long sub scapular vessels.

Central group embedded in fat in central axilla receive afferents (level 2) apical group (level 3) is found in space between pectoralis minor and clavicle and covered by clavipectoral fascia. Level 1–low axilla-lateral border of pectoralis, level 2–axilla-around pectoralis minor, level 3–apical-adjacent to axillary vein.

DEVELOPMENT ANOMALIES

- Absence of nipple athelia
- Absence of breast amazia
- Multiple nipple.

Bleeding from nipples is an expression of dysplasia-reveals blood in single segment–intraductal papilloma and duct ectasia.

Masses in Breast

Inflammatory

1. Noninfection:
   a. Traumatic
      - Injury may produce fat necrosis
      - Seen in obese women with large pendulous breast.
   b. Mammary duct ectasia
      - Common in women in sixth or seventh decade.
      - Dilatation of ducts with cell debris green in color.

c. Galactocele
   - Simple milk retension cyst, with watery and viscous discharge
   - Retension within lactiferous duct
   - Treatment chlorpromazine

2. Infection:
   a. Acute pyogenic mastitis
      - Seen in lactating women
      - Clinically breast becomes tender, red and fluctuant caused by *Staphylococcus aureas*.
      - Treatment is drainage, cloxicillin is drug of choice.

   b. Mammary tuberculosis

      Arises from haematogenous infection, leads to tuberculosis is bluish and undermined.

   c. Mammary dysplasia
      - Commonest clinical and pathological lesion of breast also called fibrocystic disease.
      - Hormonal changes occurs in women between 40–50 yrs of age.
      - Ill-defined lump in breast common in upper outer quadrant danazol for monoclonal mastalgia.
      - Ultrasound guided needle aspiration or excision.

   d. Fibroadenomas:
      - Well-circumscribed, nodules consisting of epithelial and stomach elements also called breast mouse.
      - Giant fibroadenoma called cystosarcoma phyllodes.

   e. Intraductal papilloma

      Large ducts or lactiferous sinuses and treatment is excision.

Carcinoma Breast

One out of 10 women develop breast cancer

- Risk factors include previous cancer in opposite breast, close blood relative with breast cancer, early menarche and late menopause and late first pregnancy.
- Ductal carcinoma
  a. Carcinoma *in situ*
  b. Comedo
  c. Pagets : Intraductal, ulcerated nipple and hyperchromatic cells
  d. Medullary : 15%, seen in well-formed breasts and well-differentiated gland formation
  e. Colloid : Production of mucin, intracellular and extracellular
  f. Tubular
  g. Schirous (infiltrating ductal) : Common, 60–75% and hard lump

- Diagnosis is firm, non-tender mass, having peu de orange, nipple retraction and axillary nodes.
- Mammography shows asymmetric density with microcalcification
- FNAC or biopsy

TNM classification

T_{IS} CA *in situ*
T_1 Tumor <2 cm
T_2 Tumor 2–5 cm
T_3 Tumor 5–10 cm
T_4 Tumor >10 cm
N_1 Mobile ipsilateral lymph nodes
N_2 Ipsilateral supraclavicular, mammary nodes
N_3 Ipsilateral internal mammary lymph nodes
M_1 Metastasis

Assessment includes history and examination

Below 40 years	:	Ultrasound
Above 40 years	:	Mammography
MRI	:	Impalpable breast lump

Staging

TNM

- Stage I–Tumour < 2 cm, no nodes, no metastasis
- Stage II–Tumour > 2 cm + nodes + no metastasis
- Stage III–Tumour > 5 cm + nodes + no metastasis
- Stages IV–Locally advanced + nodes + metastasis.

Other classification are Manchester, and pragmatic classification

Receptors are lob1, lob2, lob3, lob4–her-2, neureceptor membrane tyrosine in 50% cases.

Investigation done for carcinoma breast are FNAC, mammography, chest X-ray, ultrasound abdomen, estrogen receptor, progesterone receptor.

Surgery done are modified radical mastectomy and radical mastectomy.

Sentinal lymph node biopsy is done in early breast cancer without clinical palpable nodes. Preoperative injection of blue in subdermal plexus around nipple and visualized as blue staining and with a gamma camera.

Treatment

- Management of early breast cancer is controversial with recent emphasis on conservative treatment. Tumours with less than 1 cm and grade 1 tumours with less than 3 cm should be axillary clearance. For patients of ductal carcinoma *in situ* wide excision is done.
- For stage I and II segmentectomy

Followed with chest wall radiation is offered as radiation reduce risk of local recurrences in ductal carcinoma and early breast cancers.

- Classical radical mastectomy removes pectoralis major and minor muscles
- Premenopausal women with ER, PR tumours benefits from antiestrogen therapy and oophorectomy
- Older women may be given 20 mg/day
- Locally advanced breast cancer has neoadjuvant chemotherapy, radiotherapy and hormonal therapy
- Chemotherapy involves 6 cycles of CHF of cyclophosphamide, methotrexate and 5-fluorouracil
- Detection of distant metastasis is by scintigraphy, plasma calcibomin and urinary hydrostatine estimation.

  1st line : Cyclophosphamide, adriamycin, 5-fluorouracil
  2nd line : Paclitaxel, docetaxel
  3rd line : Gemcitabine

Types of Surgery

- Local wide excision
- Quadrantectomy
- Total mastectomy
- Patey mastectomy
- Radical mastectomy
- Breast conservation surgery
- Tumor 2 cm removed with skin
- Quadrant containing tumor removed
- Entire breast tissue removed
- Axillary clearance
- Breast tissue, mastectomy and pectoralis minor removed
- Entire breast tissue and pectoralis.

Muscle Removed

Survical Results

Nodes negative–10 yrs survival–78%. Nodes positive–25–48%–10 yrs survival.

Lobular Carcinoma

- Rare, found on incidental findings, 25% bilateral
- Treatment is mastectomy with biopsy of opposite side.

Prevention

- Physical examination at monthly intervals by patients and by physician at yearly intervals
- Mammography every 2 years between 35–50 years and every year after 50.

QUESTIONS AND ANSWERS

1. **How common is breast cancer? Who gets breast cancer?**
Ans: Breast cancer is the most common form of cancer in women. Women are certainly at an increased risk compared men with male breast cancer accounting for only, 1 % of all cancer breast cancers; age is also important factor. Cancer in women under 20 are very rare, but increase with age, rising slowly after/the age of 50. There is also a strong familial correlation to developing breast cancer; women whose mother's had breast cancer have 3 times the risk of the general population. Overall 1 in 10 women will have breast cancer sometimes in their life.
2. **What other tests might influence, the treatment should these tests be obtained prior to needle aspiration or biopsy?**
Ans: Mammography would be useful because may show other areas within the same breast that are suggestive of another carcinoma and it can be used to evaluate the breast. While positive mammographic findings in the same or opposite, breast may influence the treatment plan, it is important to realize that a negative mammogram does not rule out malignancy. Any suspious palpable lesion warrants biopsy whether seen on mammogram or not.
Additionally, the timings of the mammogram depends on the situation and the type of biopsy to be undertaken. An fine needle aspiration can be performed easily in the clinic, to a mammogram, without altering the mammography findings. However, mammography should always be performed prior to any open surgically biopsy.
3. **What is the next step in the workup?**
Ans: Fine needle aspiration (FNA) of the lesions is an excellent option because a diagnosis of carcinoma could be obtained prior to any surgical procedure. However, interpretations of tissue obtained from a fine needle aspiration requires a skillful cytopathologist for accurate diagnosis. A definitively positive FNA diagnosis of carcinoma would allow a final path for surgical treatment to be made without a surgical biopsy: An equivocal FNA result may require a confirmation by surgical biopsy before either the surgeon or the patient undertakes more extensive treatment. Also it is important to realize that a negative FNA biopsy not rule out a malignancy. Similar to mammography, there is a well-defined false negative rate for FNA biopsies. Any suspicious lesion with a negative FNA still warrants an excisional biopsy.
If an excisional biopsy is undertaken when the lesion is suspected to be cancerous, a excision with an attempt to obtain pathologically free margins is appropriate. The biopsy of a small lesion, as seen in this patient, may severe as a lumpectomy if all margins are clear.
A fine needle aspiration was performed and was " highly suspicious" for carcinoma.
4. **What are the treatment options?**
Ans: The term " highly suspicious" imply some level of doubt on the part of the pathologist if there is any doubt, and biopsy should be performed prior to operative treatment. If the diagnosis is definitive, surgical treatment may follow.
Several well designed studies have shown that segmental mastectomy (lumpectomy) coupled with axillary node dissection and radiation therapy, is equivalent to modified radical mastectomy.
Level 1: Axillary lymph nodes lateral to pectoralis minor
Level 2: Posterior to pectoralis minor
Level 3: Medial to pectoralis minor

5. **What are nerves encountered in axillary dissection?**
Ans: Long thoracic nerve innervates serratus anterior thoracodorsal nerve innervates lattismus dorsi.
6. **What is difference between modified radical mastectomy and radical mastectomy?**
Ans: Surgeons remove breast, pectoral fascia and axillary node as modified radical mastectomy.
Stage 1 : 60–80%
Stage 2 : 30–45%
Radical mastectomy removes breast, pectoral fascia, axillary lymph nodes and pectoralis major.
7. **What are commonest histologic types of breast cancer?**
Ans: Commonest histological type of breast is infiltrating ductal carcinoma.
8. **When do you give chemotherapy?**
Ans: A. Premenopausal women
Node positive–Adjuvant chemotherapy
B. Premenopausal women
Node negative–No further therapy
C. Premenopausal
Node negative–No further therapy
D. Premenopausal
ER, PR Receptors–Adjuvant
Positive–Tamoxifen is oestogen receptor antagonist.
9. **What is fibrocystic disease of breast and treatment?**
Ans: Patients with fibrocystic disease have pain, swelling, tenderness, nodularity during menstruation treatment is by analgesics, vitamins, danazol.
10. **What is hormonal therapy for carcinoma breast?**
Ans: Premenopausal
Tamoxifen–Antiestrogen
Progesteron–Medroxy Progesterone 400 mg
Postmenopausal
Tamoxifen
Aromatase inhibitor like Letrozole 2.5 mg o.d. monoclonal antibody transtuzumab (herceptin her-2 acts on herz receptors
Progestogens
Androgens
Medical adrenalectomy using aminoglutethemide (mitotane)
Oophorectomy

Flow Chart: Breast cancer

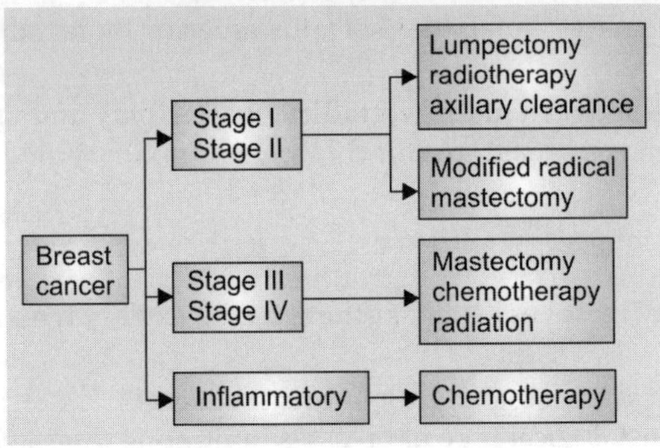

Flow Chart: Lump breast

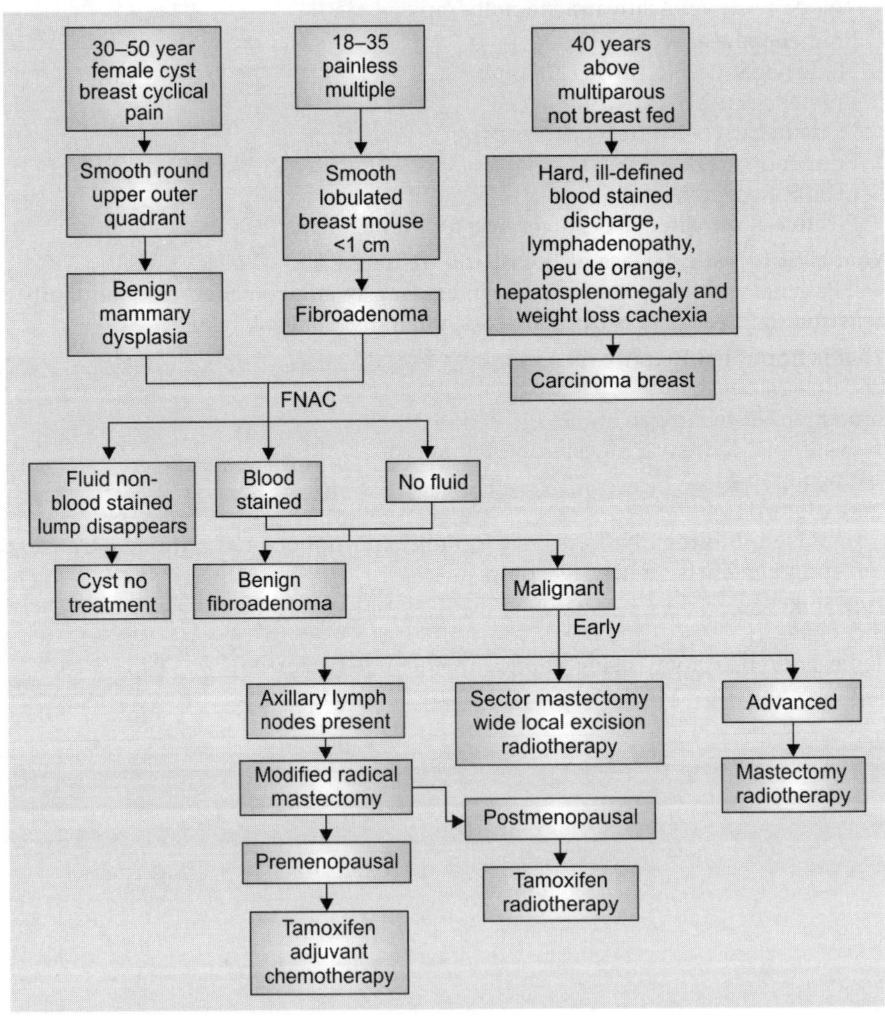

Flow Chart: Breast cancer treatment

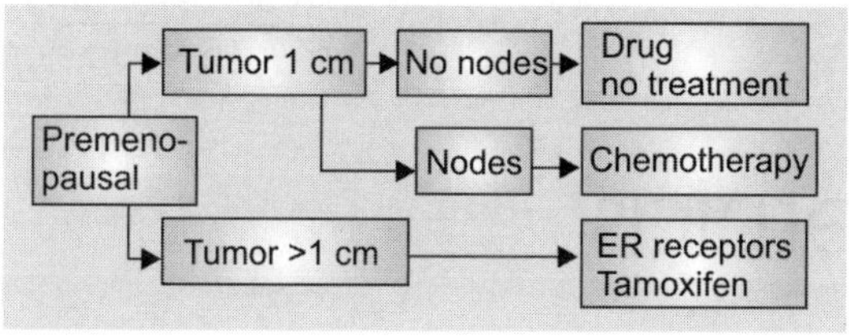

Flow Chart: Breast pain

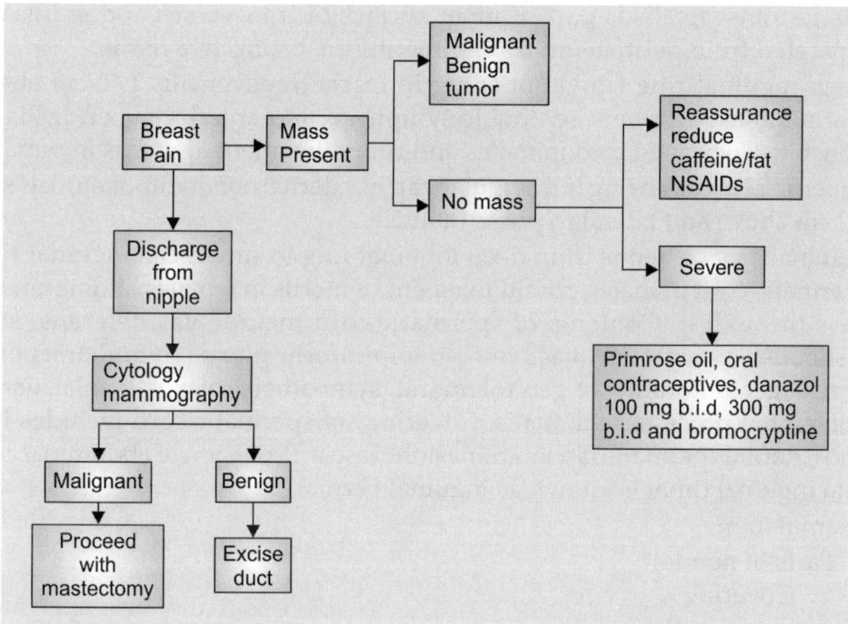

9

Hernias

ANATOMY

Hernias is defined as abnormal protrusion of viscous or part of viscous through opening with a sac covering it.

A. Fascia transversalis is part of inner surface of transversus abdominis muscle separated from peritoneum by extraperitoneal connective tissue.
B. Deep inguinal ring is oval opening in fascia transversalis 1/2 cm above the midinguinal point between pubic symphysis and anterior superior iliac spine transmits spermatic cord in males and round ligament of uterus in females.
C. Superficial inguinal ring is triangular gap in external oblique aponeurosis situated 1.2 cm above and lateral to pubic tubercle.
D. Inguinal canal extends from deep inguinal ring to superficial inguinal ring and spermatic cord in males, round ligament of uterus in females, ilioinguinal nerve pass through it. Contents of spermatic cord include vas deferens, arteries-testicular, cremasteric, vas, veins-pampiniform plexus, lymphatics of testis, nerves-genital branch of genitofemoral, sympathetic plexus-areolar tissue and obliterated processus vaginalis. Coverings of spermatic cord includes internal and external spermatic fascia, cremasteric fascia. Protusion of abdominal contents into inguinal canal is known as inguinal hernia.
E. Examination:
   1. Parts of hernia
      a. Covering
      b. Sac
      c. Contents
   2. Differential diagnosis of groin lump include inguinal, femoral, saphena varix, aneurysms, skin lumps, psoas abscess and ectopic testis.
      a. Can you get above swelling
      b. Is it separate from testis
      c. Is it cystic or solid
         - Separate and cystic–epididymal cyst
            - Separate and solid–epididymitis
            - Testicular and cystic–hydrocele
            - Testicular and solid–tumor and orchitis
      d. In cough impulse present or not
      e. Ultrasound may be used to differentiate from tumors.

Epididymal cysts–develops in adult life, has clear or milky spermatocoele fluid and lie above testis.

Hydrocele–fluid within tunica vaginalis associated with patent processus vaginalis.

Epididymitis–causes include Chlamydia, *E. coli,* mumps, gonococcal. Take a urine sample and look for discharge.

Classification of Hernia

Type 1: Hernia has tight internal ring through which peritoneal sac passes out as indirect sac

Type 2: Hernia has moderately enlarged ring and once reduced hernia protrudes on coughing and straining

Type 3: Hernia has large internal ring and once reduced it protrudes without straining

Type 4: Direct hernia with defect of posterior wall ring

Type 5: Direct hernia protruding from defect in fascia transversalis

Type 6: Pantaloon hernia

Type 7: Femoral hernia.

GROIN HERNIAS

Indirect Hernia

1. These result from a persistent patent processus vaginalis and thus are considered congenital in origin, although they may not become manifest until later in life.
2. Hernia contents descend through the internal ring to the inferior epigastric vessels, descend down the spermatic cord toward and sometimes into the scrotum.
3. The most common type of hernia in any age or sex group.
4. Development in elderly ages may be associated with COPD and chronic cough, straining on urination due to prostatic disease, straining on defecation due to colonic disease (including colon cancers).
5. Recurrence rate with first time repair is 2.5–5%, this increase with each subsequent repair.

Direct Hernia

1. Associated with defect in the fascia of the floor of the inguinal canal–Hesselbach's triangle bounded by the rectus sheath medially and superiorly inguinal ligament inferiorly and the inferior epigastric vessels laterally.
2. Less commonly associated with incarceration or strangulation.
3. Associated with chronic use and significant strain on muscle and fascia layers, including, COPD, BHP and colon cancer.

Treatment

1. Operation is the treatment of choice and may be performed using general, local, epidural or spinal analgesia.

2. All childhood hernias are indirect and a herniotomy is performed. This operation is the ligation of the sac. In the adult with an indirect hernia the posterior wall of the inguinal canal is repaired addition-herniorrhaphy. If the hernia is direct and there is therefore no indirect sac, herniorrhaphy alone is performed.
3. A reducible hernia in an adult should ideally be repaired by herniorrhaphy. Any enlarging hernia, with time, may become irreducible. This is itself is not an indication for urgent surgery, but if symptoms of obstruction or ischaemia accompany it then immediate surgical intervention is required.
4. Repair usually involves reduction of Hernia Mass with tight closure of the internal ring and repair of the floor of the canal by Bassini method, shouldice repair meshplasty (Lichenstein) repair, Laparoscopic Total Extraperitoneal (TEP) repair, Trans Abdominal Preperitoneal (TAPP) repair is popular choice for repair of bilateral and recurrent inguinal hernias.

Femoral Hernia

1. Herniation of the intra-abdominal contents through the femoral canal bounded laterally by the femoral vein, anteriorly by the inguinal ligament, posteriorly by the rim of the pubis.
2. More common in women than in men.
3. Felt to have an increased incidence of incarceration or strangulation.
4. Repair requires suprainguinal ligament repair.

Complications

1. Incarceration–indicates inability of the hernia contents to be reduced to their normal position.
2. Strangulation–indicates occlusion of the vascular supply to the hernia contents and results in much greater morbidity and mortality.

Examination of Groin Hernias

Expansile impulse on coughing over swelling is diagnostic. It is better seen than felt. Contents are reduced on lying down and by direct pressure.

Expansile impulse is seen in standing position. Deep ring occlusion test is when deep using is occluded after reducing contents, if impulse on coughing is absent then it is indirect inguinal hernia.

Zieman test is done for knowing what type of hernia when superficial ring, deep ring and femoral ring is occluded.

Finger invagination test is done and impulse felt on superficial ring whether it is at tip or and pulp. Palpation of testis, epididymis and spermatic cord should be done.

Sliding hernias: Part of wall of hernias is an intra-abdominal content of right side most commonly colon, left side may be bladder. In females this involves anomalies.

Richter hernia: Involves incarceration of wall of hernia in hernia opening leading to necrosis.

Ventral hernias: Any protrusions through abdominal wall are defined as ventral hernias.

Umbilical hernias: Most commonly occurring in young children resolve by age of two. This is herniation through an umbilical scar. Presents with swelling in umbilical regions. Indications for surgery are if persists after age of two years and defect more than 2 cm. Surgery is by infraumbilical incision sac identified and ligated by transfixation. Defect is closed with interrupted nonabsorbable sutures.

Paraumbilical hernias: Occurs in adults. Protrusion of hernia through linea alba above and below the umbilicus.

Mayo operation by transverse incisions sac is dissected. Herniotomy is done. Double breasting of defect can also be done. Meshplasty can be done in larger umbilical and paraumbilical hernias whereas after reduction of sac and closure of defect, mesh is placed on the sheath. Umbilectomy may be required.

Epigastric hernias: It occurs through defect in linea alba between xiphoid and umbilicus. Clinical features are pain and swelling in epigastric region. Treatment is by mayo repair and meshplasty.

Incisional hernias: These occur after precious operative procedures usually result of wound infection, necrosis of fascia, breakage of sutures, presence of tuberculosis, jaundice, anaemia and malignancy. Clinical feature are swelling in scar region and impulse on coughing. Defect is felt and assessed.

Catells repair of hernia can be done when defect is less than 3 cm. Double breasting and meshplasty done. Laparoscopic repair of incisional hernias can be done by placing mesh after reducing abdominal contents from defect. Intraperitoneal onlay mesh is put and mesh is fixed with tackers.

Other types of ventral hernias include spigelian hernia which is herniation at semilunar line of Douglas and Petit triangle hernia where hernia is from inferior lumbar triangle posteriorly.

QUESTIONS AND ANSWERS

1. **Define hernia**
   Ans: Abnormal protrusion of viscous or part of viscous through an opening with a sac covering it.
2. **What are types of hernias?**
   Ans: Incidence of hernias are inguinal indirect 5%, direct 25%, femoral 16%, incisional 10%, umbilical 3%, others 3%.
3. **What is incarcerated hernias?**
   Ans: A hernia is incarcerated when contents of sac cannot be reduced into abdomen and part of wall of bowel may be necrosed.
4. **What is sliding internal hernia?**
   Ans: Sliding hernia is when one layer of hernia sac is made of bowel.
5. **Petit's hernia**
   Ans: (Rare) hernia through Petit's triangle (AKA inferior lumbar triangle) (think: Petit = small = inferior).

6. **Grynfeltt's hernia**
Ans: Hernia through Grynfeltt-Lesshaft triangle (superior lumbar triangle).
7. **Pantaloon hernia**
Ans: Hernia sac exists as both a direct and indirect hernia protruding through the floor of the canal as well as the internal ring (two sac separated by the inferior epigastric vessels).
8. **Richter's hernia**
Ans: Incarcerated or strangulated hernia involving only one sidewall of the bowel, which can spontaneously reduce, resulting in gangrenous bowel and perforation within the abdomen without signs of obstruction.
9. **Morgagni's hernia**
Ans: Anterior parasternal diaphragmatic hernia.
10. **Bassini**
Ans: Sutures approximate reflection of inguinal ligament (Poupart's) to the transversus abdominis aponeurosis/conjoint tendon
11. **Lichenstein**
Ans: "Tension-free" repair using mesh.
12. **Shouldice**
Ans: Imbrication of the floor of the inguinal canal (AKA "Canadian repair").
13. **Plug and Patch**
Ans: Placing a plug of mesh in hernia defect and then overlaying a patch of mesh over inguinal floor (requires few if any sutures in mesh!).
14. **High ligation**
Ans: Ligation and transaction of indirect hernia sac with repair of inguinal floor (used only in children).
15. **TAPP procedure**
Ans: Trans abdominal pre peritoneal inguinal hernia repair.
16. **TEP procedure**
Ans: Totally extra peritoneal repair.
17. **What are the indications for laparoscopic inguinal hernia repair?**
   a. Bilateral inguinal hernia
   b. Recurrent hernia.
18. **What is first subcutaneous named layer?**
Ans: Scarpa's fascia.
19. **What is the name of the subcutaneous vein that is ligated?**
Ans: Superficial epigastric vein.
20. **What happens if you cut the illioinguinal nerve?**
Ans: Numbness of inner thigh or lateral scrotum; usually goes away in 6 months.
21. **From what abdominal muscle layer is the cremaster muscle derived?**
Ans: Internal oblique muscle.
22. **To what does the inguinal (Poupart's) ligament attach?**
Ans: Anterior superior iliac spine to the public tubercle.
23. **What is the hernia sac made of?**
Ans: Basically peritoneum or a patent processus vaginalis.

24. What is Hesselbach's triangle?
   a. Epigastric vessels
   b. Inguinal ligament
   c. Lateral border of the rectus sheath.

25. What is a relaxing incision?
Ans: "Incision(s) in the rectus sheath to relax the conjoint tendon so that it can be approximated to the reflection of the inguinal ligament without tension.

26. What is the conjoint tendon?
Ans: The aponeurotic attachments of the transversus abdominis to the pubic tubercle.

27. What is the boundary of the femoral canal?
   a. Cooper's ligament posteriorly
   b. Inguinal ligament anteriorly
   c. Femoral vein laterally
   d. Lacunar ligament medially.

28. What is the Howship-Romberg sign?
Ans: Pain along the medial aspect of the proximal thigh from nerve compression caused by obturator hernia.

29. What is the silk glove sign?
Ans: The inguinal hernia sac in an infant/toddler feels like a finger of a silk glove when rolled under the examining finger.

Flow Chart: Scrotal lumps

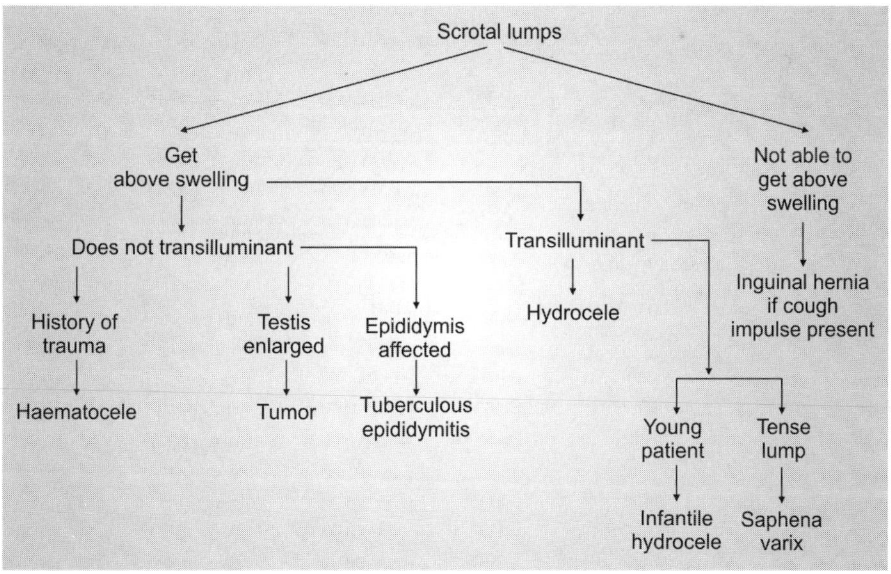

Flow Chart

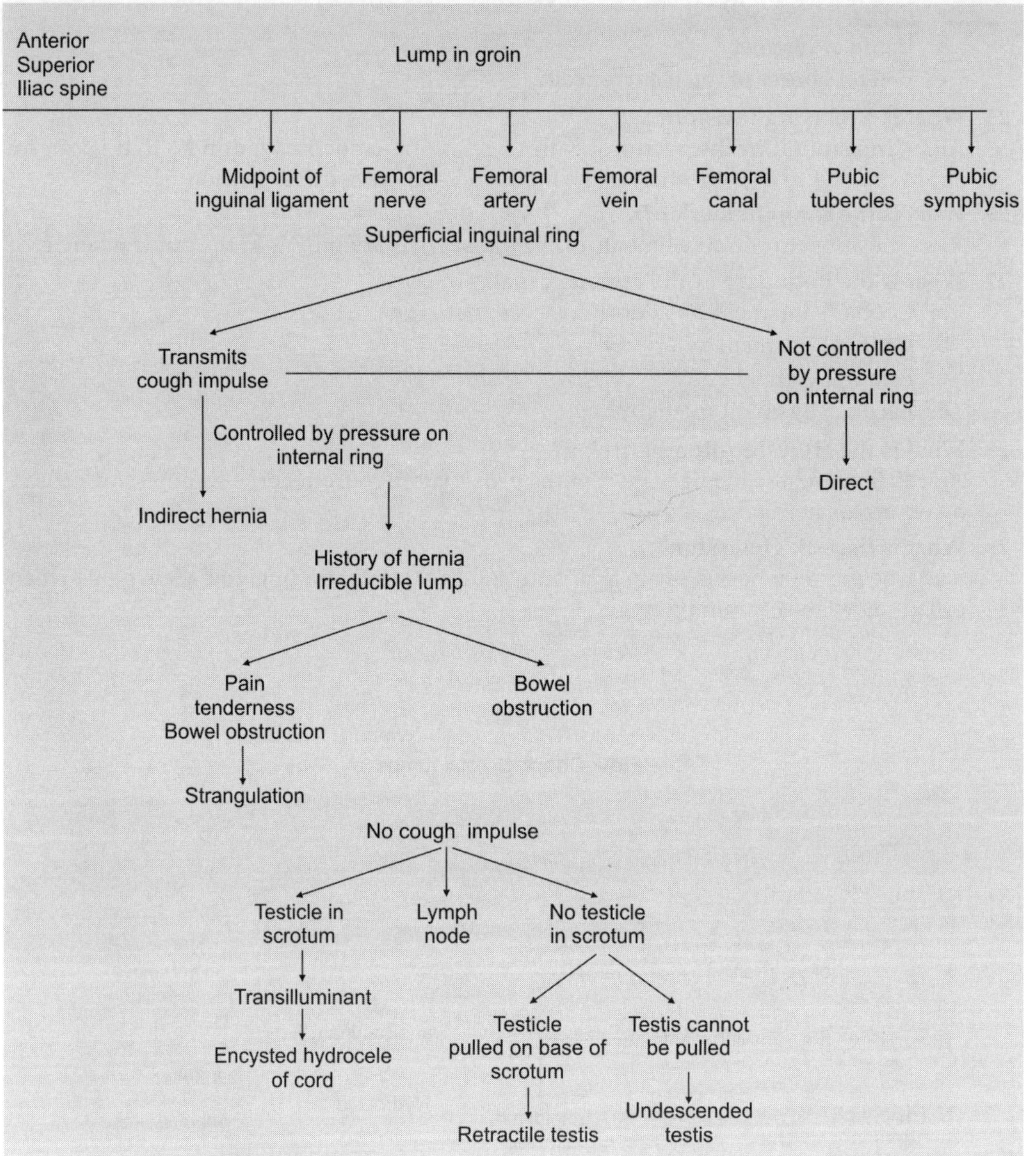
Anterior
Superior
Iliac spine
Lump in groin
Midpoint of
inguinal ligament
Femoral
nerve
Femoral
artery
Femoral
vein
Femoral
canal
Pubic
tubercles
Pubic
symphysis
Superficial inguinal ring
Transmits
cough impulse
Not controlled
by pressure
on internal ring
Controlled by pressure on
internal ring
Direct
Indirect hernia
History of hernia
Irreducible lump
Pain
tenderness
Bowel obstruction
Bowel
obstruction
Strangulation
No cough impulse
Testicle in
scrotum
Lymph
node
No testicle
in scrotum
Transilluminant
Testicle
pulled on base of
scrotum
Testis cannot
be pulled
Encysted hydrocele
of cord
Undescended
testis
Retractile testis

10

Endocrine

ANATOMY

Thyroid glands develop from pharyngeal floor between 1st and 2nd pharynageal Pouches. The canalised column becomes thyroglossal duct which forms thyroid lobes.

1. Follicles with supporting stroma and parafollicular cells (C cells).
2. Right, left lobe and isthmus extends past hyoid bone to foremen caecum at base of tongue.
3. Arterial supply–inferior thyroid artery branches of thyrocervical trunk and superior thyroid arteries branches of external carotid are inferior, middle and superior.
4. External laryngeal nerve runs with superior thyroid artery recurrent laryngeal nerve loops around aortic arch on left, subclavian artery on right usually bends near thyrocervical groove, behind inferior thyroid artery to enter larynx.

PHYSIOLOGY

1. Serum iodine converted to T_3 and T_4 which have different effects on organs.
2. Parafollicular also secrete calcitonin, which regulates calcium levels.

LUMPS IN THE THYROID

Examination: Watch the neck during swallowing water. Stand behind and feel thyroid for size, shape (smooth? One or many nodules?). Tenderness and mobility. Percuss for retrosternal extension. Any nodes? Bruits? If this enlarged (goitre), ask these 3 questions:

1. If the thyroid smooth or nodular?
2. Is the patient euthyroid, thyrotoxic or hypothyroid, smooth, nontoxic, goiter? Endemic (iodine deficiency); congenital; goiter-gens; thyroiditis, physiological Hashimoto's thyroiditis (an autoimmune disease thought to be due to apoptosis induced by lymphocytes combining with thyrocytes. Smooth, toxic, goiter: Graves disease.
3. Any nodules. Many or one. If >4 cm across, malignancy is more likely. Multinodular goiter usually euthyroid but hyperthyroidism may develop. Hypothyroidism and malignancy are rare.

The single thyroid lump is a common problem 10% will be malignant. Causes: Cyst, adenoma, discrete nodule in multinodular goiter, malignancy. First ask is he/she thyrotoxic? Do T_3 and T_4 then, ultrasound, to see if the lump is solid or cystic or part of a group of lumps. Fine-needle aspiration (FNA) and to do cytology on the fluid. No clinical or lab test is good enough to tell for sure if follicular neoplasms identified on FNA are benign, so most such patient are referred for surgery.

METHODS OF INVESTIGATION OF THE THYROID

1. Mechanical effect
   a. Clinically–degree of stridor
   b. Radiographically–air or contrast laryngography and tracheography
   c. Endoscopically
2. Sites of activity
   a. Scanning or gamma camera pictures of areas of radioactive iodine uptake.
3. Function
   i. Basal-metabolic rate: Measurement of energy output under resting conditions by measuring the oxygen uptake and standardizing the result with reference to surface area. An investigation which is difficult technically and prone to many inaccuracies.
   ii. Blood cholesterol: A presumptive diagnosis of hypothyroidism is made if the level is over 8 mmol/1 (300 mg/100 ml) if other causes of hypercholesterolaemia may be excluded.
   iii. Protein bound iodine: Measures bounds thyroid hormone levels but is prone to inaccuracy from ingested or administered iodine compounds, especially contrast media, and from variation in the binding glubin levels. Normal level 280 to 630 nmol/1 (3.5 to 8.4 mg/100 ml).
   iv. ^{131}I uptake test: Tends to be inaccurate because of other interactions. Require multiple measurements in a specialist laboratory over 2 days. Normal uptake 20 to 55 % in 24 hours. Plasma clearance 5 to 60 ml/min.
   v. ^{131}I uptake, ^{99}mTc uptake: Both used because of the lower radiation at the gland. Normal uptake less than 3% at 20 min.

Thyroid Nodules

1. It is the commonest presentation of thyroid cancer and are malignant in 10% cases. History of irradiation increases malignancy by 30–50%. Thyroid cancer in cervical node metasis is called lateral abberent thyroid.
2. History of hormones, pain, shortness of branch, explosure to radiation, family history, MEN syndromes followed by clinical examination, FNAC, ultrasound CT scan and MRI thyroid scans, thyroid function test.

Thyroid Tumours

Benign Tumours

Follicular adenoma may be differentiated by absence of capsular or vascular invasion. The hurthle cell adenoma contains large acidophilic granular cells with minimal signs of follicular with little colloid. Treatment are present in young adults, rare, and presence of calcification is diagnostic.

Solitary Thyroid Nodule

Nodules diagnosed clinically are found to be multiple in 50% cases at surgery or histology.

Pathology

1. Clinically toxic patients usually have a simple adenoma but these form a small group; about 6% of cases.
2. The incidence of malignancy is quoted between 6% and 58% (nodular goitre 1% to 25%) but in most series at 6% to 12%.

Investigation

1. Blood investigation for thyrotoxicosis.
2. Soft tissue radiographs of the neck to detect any tracheal compression.
3. Isotopic scanning is of little value since both 'cold' and 'warm' nodules have an incidence of malignancy (12.8% and 6% respectively).
4. Lymphography
5. Needle biopsy
6. High-speed drill biopsy can be useful.

Management

1. *Exploration and nodulectomy with wide clearance:* Hemithyriodectomy–carefully preserve the recurrent laryngeal nerve and parathyroid with blood supply. This technique ensures clearance of the tumour but with little morbidity. Taking the whole isthmus ensures that no problems arise from compression when the remainder hypertrophies. Frozen section is only recommended for suspicious carcinoma.
2. Total thyroidectomy for clinically unequivocal carcinoma.
3. Papillary carcinoma accounts for 60–80% of all thyroid carcinomas, mixed papillary or follicular. Capsular invasions, in present, spread young age groups. Tumours are multifocal, bilateral 50% spread to lymph nodes. Spread could be metasis and local invasion. Treatment is total thyroidectomy. Suppressive doses of thyroxine are given all cases of total thyroidectomy and hormones sensitive.
4. Follicular carcinoma accounts for 10–18% thyroid cancer, single, encapsulated, 3 cm in diameter. Prognosis depends on vascular invasion occurs in fifth and sixth decade and metastases to bone and lung. Radioactive iodine treatment of choice.
5. Iduratile cell tumours are variants of follicular, tumours and made thyroid, lymphatics and regional lymph nodes. Total thyroidectomy is recommended and radioactive iodine is of little help.
6. Medullary carcinoma accounts for 5–10% of all thyroid neoplasms. Sporadic 80% and MEN syndrome in 20%. Tumour of parafollicular cells which secrete

calcitonin. MEN II-A autosomal dominant with MTC and parathyroid neoplasms. Treatment is total thyroidectomy and dissection of anterior compartment of neck. MEN II-B phaechromocytoma, marfanoid tumour, multiple neuromas and medullary carcinomas.

7. Anaplastic carcinomas accounts for 5–14% of primary neoplasms characterized by rapid growth, tissue infiltration, seventh decade, trachea compression and cervical lymphadenopathy and recurrent nerve paresis is visible. Treatment is radiotherapy. Malignant lymphoma common in sixth decade, females, majority are B-cell Hodgkin's and treatment is chemotherapy and radiotherapy.

Indications

Pressure symptoms, hyperthyroid and carcinoma.

Treatment

1. Papillary and follicular tumors
   a. Extra capsular thyroidectomy preserving the parathyroids and their blood supply. Frozen section may be necessary for sections of enlarged lymph nodes be necessary for sections of enlarged lymph nodes. If tumors are found then a local lymph node resection is adequate and radical block dissection need not be done.
   b. Postoperatively a diagnostic scan is performed and if locally activity is found a therapeutic dose of ^{131}I is given (about 200 mCi).
   c. Inoperable cases are treated with ^{131}I if functioning or with external irradiation with high energy beams. Secondary may be treated similarly.
2. Anaplastic tumors
   a. Total thyroidectomy
   b. Postoperative irradiation to the neck and upper mediastinum
   c. Inoperative tumors are irradiated.
3. Medullary tumors
   a. Total thyroidectomy
   b. Irradiation for residual tumor or for inoperable tumor.
4. Lymphomas

   These are treated like lymphomas elsewhere by biopsy and irradiation including the upper mediastinum in the field.

Hormone Therapy

Well differentiated tumors in childhood may be TSH dependent and regress if thyroid hormones are administered. Thyroid hormones are given routinely following thyroidectomy; hormone therapy alone is not employed.

Chemotherapy

Chemotherapy may be especially useful in lymphomas. In tumors other than lymphomas it has little part to play at present.

Complications

Recurrent laryngeal nerve palsy, haemorrhage, hypothyroidism, thyroid storm (treat by propanol, antithyroid drugs + iodine) and hyperparathyroidism.

THYROID CANCER

A. Thyroid cancer
   Comprises 0.7% of all malignancies in men and 0.2% in women.
B. A etiology
   1. Endemic goiter is thought to predispose to thyroid cancer, due to the raised TSH level. This has been proved in animals but the statistics in man are mixed.
   2. Irradiation, especially at low levels in children, raises the incidence. There may be a 20-year or more latent period.
   3. Some forms of medullary carcinomas are familial.
C. Pathology
   1. Tumours derived from follicular cells may be:
      a. Largely follicular
      b. Largely papillary
      c. Anaplastic
   2. Tumours derived from parafollicular cells are medullary.
   3. Lymphomas may present in the thyroid.
D. Incidence
   1. Papillary 48%
   2. Follicular 20%
   3. Anaplastic 25%
   4. Medullary 7%
E. Clinical features
   1. May present with diffuse swelling, nodular swelling or single nodule. Occasionally presents with lymph node involvement or secondary metastases.
   2. Presence of hoarseness or Horner's syndrome signify extracapular spread and worse prognosis.
   3. Patients under 30 years tend to have a papillary carcinoma with a good prognosis. Over 50% 10-year-survival.

MULTINODULAR GOITRE

A. Multinodular goitre
   Hyperfunctioning of thyroid gland leading to thyrotoxicosis. Subtotal thyroidectomy with thyroxine replacements given later.
B. Thyrotoxicosis
   1. Grave disease
   2. Toxic multinodular goiter
   3. Toxic nodules

It affect young females, symptoms are weight loss, heat intolerance, tremor, anxiety, diarrhoea and menstrual irregularity. Signs are exophthalmos, lid lag, tachycardia, ophthalmoplegia. Treatment is carbimazole 15 mg.

Complications presents with diabetes, skin rash elevated serum glucagon, localized by CT and angiography. Venous thromboembolism and malignancy may be present. Palliation is by somatostatin.

Vipoma is a neuroendocrine tumour which secretes vasoactive intestinal polypeptide (VIP). Presentation is triad of watery diarrhea, hypokalemia, achlorrhydria. Diagnosis is done by serum VIP, CT, selective angiography. Treatments is correction and electrolyte imbalance and subtotal pancreatectomy.

C. Inflammatory goiter
   1. Hashimotos disease diffuse inflammation with antibiotics against thyroglobulin, midline aged female presenting with goiter, enlarged T_4 50–200 µg/day, thyroidectomy required occasionally.
   2. Dequervains–thyroiditis in non suppurative inflammation due to cox virus presents with swollen, tender gland preceded by sorethroat. Management is prednisolone 10–20 mg.
   3. Reider's thyroiditis is recurrent laryngeal nerve palsy, stridor. Treatment is T_4 hormone.

D. Pancreatic tumours of endocrine origin
   Rare <1 in 100,000 most prevalent is:
   1. Insulinoma which solitary benign unless associated with MEN I. There is whipple triad
      a. Signs and symptoms of hypocalcaemia during fasting
      b. At time of symptoms blood sugar level is 50 mg/dl
      c. Symptom are reversed by intravenous administration of glucose.
      Diagnosis is fasting insulin levels compared with glucose. Normal <0.35. Distal pancreatectomy for malignant lesions. Subtotal pancreatectomy for MEN I associated tumours
      d. Gastronoma or Zollinger-Ellision syndrome results of gastric hypersecretion and peptic ulcer alone associated with 80–90% are around head of pancreas. Treatment is with steptoztocin.
      Radioiodine is reversed for patients are 40 years of age, recurrent thyrotoxicosis following subtotal thyroidectomy.
      Carcinoid tumours arise from enterochromaffin cells which sites are appendix (45%), ileum (30%), large gut 20%, lung and bronchus 10%. Tumours >2 cm are clinically malignant. Diagnosis is twenty four hour urinary 5-hydroxyindole acetic acid (5-HIAA), and monoclonal antibody isotype scanning. Carcinoid syndrome is facial flushing, diarrhoea, hepatosplenomegaly, bronchoconstriction, telangiectasis of face and right sided heart failure. Treatment is somatastatin analogue and cytotoxic. Treatment of 5-FU. Surgery in certain cases is helpful.

PARATHYROID

A. Anatomy: Usually 4 glands 2 inferior ones derived from 3rd pharyngeal pouch and 2 superior ones derived from 4th pharyngeal pouch. Blood supply from branches of inferior and superior thyroid arteries.

B. Physiology
   1. Produces parathyroid hormone and maintains serum calcium between 8.5 and 10.5
   2. Hyperparathyroidism is most prevalent cause of hypercalcaemia and second commonest cause of hypercalcemia in hospitalized patients after malignancy 1:1000 and access in fifth and sixth decade. Presentations could be urinary tract calculi bone and joint pain, GI symptoms like constipation, pancreatitis, hypertension and polydypsia. Most common pathology is solitary adenoma preoperative localization is by technetium 99m ultrasound, CT scan and MRI. Excision is done with single adenoma. Inhyperplasia 3–1/2 gland removal with half gland autotransplantation into forearm. Hypocalaemia shows features of tingling sensations and spasm of feet and hands (tetany). Trousseau's sign (hypocalcaemia after cuff inflation) or Chvostek's sign (tapping of facial nerve causing tinnitus), carpopedal spasm is hand flexed at metacarpophalangeal joint with straight finger and thumb adducted, foot and toes planter flexed. Treatment is with calcium gluconate 10% in 10 ml).
   3. Treated with excision of parathyroid adenoma
   4. Overall most common cause of hypercalcemia is metastatic cancers to bones–especially from lung, breast, colon, prostate and myeloma.

C. Secondary–tertiary HPT
   1. 2° HPT occurs in renal failure patients on hemodialysis whose serum Ca^{++} is low but whose PTH level remains high. This promotes soft tissues calcification, especially in arteries.
   2. 3° HPT is diagnosed when the hemodialysis patient gets a kidney transplant which tries to regulate serum Ca^{++} level but has persistent increased PTH levels causing hypercalcemia.
      a. 3° HPT is usually associated with glands hypertrophy and is treated with either excision of 3 ½ glands of excision of all glands and reimplantation of ½ gland into a forearm muscle.

D. Parathyroid carcinoma
   1. Parathyroid is 3–6 cm in length and orange in colour
   2. Very rare–may not be associated with severely increased Ca^{++}
   3. Suspect it if a palpable tumor mass is present or the parathyroid gland does not easily dissect away from surroundings tissues.

E. Hypoparthyroidism
   1. Rare except as complication of thyroid of parathyroid surgery
   2. Treated with calcium and vitamin D supplements.

ADRENAL GLAND

1. Left side-gland juxtaposes kidney, spleen, pancreas and diaphragm
   a. Arterial supply from renal artery branches, aortic branches and phrenic branches

b. Main draining vein empties into left renal vein.
2. Right side–gland juxtaposes kidney, vena cava, liver, diaphragm
a. Arterial supply–branch of renal branches, phrenic branch
b. Vein is very short and drains into IVC.

A. Physiology
1. Responsible for wide range of mostly cholesterol-derived hormones–catecholamines, aldosterone (mineralocorticoids), glucocorticoids, estrogen, androgens, etc.

B. Pheochromocytoma–3 per million.
1. Metabolically active adenoma (only 10% are malignant) of the adrenal medulla (although 10% are in neuroendocrine rests outside the adrenal gland) that produces catecholamines norepinephrine but also epinephrine).
2. Associated with MEN II (pituitary, medullary carcinoma of thyroid, pheochromocytome) and with von Recklinghausen neurofibromatosis but most common is an isolated tumor (50–70%) 10% are unilateral but in familial cases, 50% are bilateral.
3. Usually manifestation is that of sustained high blood pressure (HBP) but the classic manifestations are those of episodic catecholamine release–bursts of tachycardia, diaphoresis, headaches, weight loss, nausea and vomiting, Raynaud's phenomenon, etc.
4. Diagnosis is by detecting VMA and metanephrine levels in urine–localizing test including CT scanning and/or iodocholestrol scans.
5. VMA >35 mmol/24 hours. Total catecholamines >1 microgram/liter. Urinary adrenaline >20 micrograms/24 hrs.
6. Treatment
a. Initial suppression of catecholamine activity–phenoxybenzamine or phentolamine–beta-blockers (propranolol) if tachycardia develops and simultaneous increasing of intravascular volume.
b. Adrenalectomy either open or laparoscopic.
Lateral approach through 11th ribs unless the tumour is big then anterior transperitoneal approach. Intraoperative hypertension crisis treated with volume expansion and antihypertensives.

C. Primary hyperaldosternoism (Conn's syndrome).
1. The most common etiology is a benign adenoma of zona glomerulosa adrenal gland. 72% benign cortical adenoma secreting aldosterone. 27% bilateral cortical hyperplasia, carcinoma is rare.
2. Manifestations include sustained hypertension (usually mild-to-moderate) with a characteristic hypokalemic metabolic alkalosis and polyuria, polydipsia and muscular weakness.
3. High serum levels of aldosterone and low levels of serum rennin are diagnostic
4. Localizing studies include CT scanning or iodocholesterol scans.
5. Treatment consists of excision of the involved adrenal gland, usually through posterior lateral laparoscopic approach.

D. Cushing's syndrome/disease

1. Cushing disease consists of adenoma of anterior pituitary gland secreting cortisol stimulating hormone (ACTH) resulting in stigmata of chronic excess glucocorticoids (60%).
2. The most common cause of Cushing's syndrome is secondary to iatrogenic administration of glucocorticoids.
   a. May also result from ectopic source of ACTH (i.e., oat cell carcinoma of lung)
   b. Adrenal adenomas or carcinomas may occasionally cause Cushing's syndrome (15%).
3. Manifestations include hypertension, central obesity, purple stria, diabetes mellitus, weakness, amenorrhea, nervousness, irritability, bone pain, osteoporosis, hirsutism, headache, ankle and hand edema, decreased libido in females and feminization of males.
4. Diagnosis started with urinary and serum cortisol levels. Dexamethasone suppression best may confirm presence of Cushing's syndrome and discriminate the syndrome from the disease.
5. Localizing efforts include CT scanning and iodocholesterol scanning after pituitary adenomas have been ruled out.
6. Treatment consists of ablation of pituitary if a tumour can be found or bilateral adrenal excision with glucocorticoids and mineralocorticoid replacement.
7. Nelson's syndrome may occur after bilateral adrenalectomy–pituitary enlargement causing visual field loss and hyperpigmentation.

E. Hypoaldosteronism (Addison's disease)

1. Hypoaldosteronism is usually secondary to infectious destruction of the adrenal gland (histoplasmosis) or trauma to the adrenal gland (hemorrhage in patients on anticoagulation or surgical removal).
2. Manifested by flucating blood pressure control and electrolyte abnormalities.
3. Treatment requires glucocorticoid and mineralocorticoid replacement.

QUESTIONS AND ANSWERS

1. **What would be your differential diagnosis of a neck mass?**
   Ans: Approximately 50% of neck masses originate from the thyroid gland. Inflammatory, nonthyroidal malignant and congenital lesions result in the remaining 50%. Malignant lesions, such as hyperparathyroid crisis. Parathyroidectomy is typically performed after the patient has improved and the diagnosis is confirmed; however, emergent operative intervention is advocated by many surgeons in the absence of a prompt response to medical therapy by the patient.
2. **Your patient has a solitary nodule palpable in the thyroid and a scan shows that it is 'hot' with suppression of the rest of the gland. Is the likely to be malignant?**
   Ans: No, It is excessively unusual for hot nodules to be malignant, they are usually benign adenomata. They should be excised by hemithyroidectomy and the prognosis is good.

3. **What instructions should be given to a patient about to commerce a course of Carbimazole for hyperparathyroidism?**
   Ans: This drug must be taken 8 hourly and not 'three times a day'. The common cause of treatment failure is irregular timing of the drug. The major (rare) side effect is bone marrow depression. Ask the patient to report any sore throats or malaise, and do an F.B.C. blood sugar test.
4. **What ENT investigation should usually be performed prior to any thyroid operation?**
   Ans: Indirect laryngoscopy (an outpatient procedure). Up to 3% of the population have an asymptomatic partial or complete cord palsy. If any Question of operative recurrent laryngeal nerve damage arises, this base-line information may be of great value.
5. **Why are preoperative X-rays taken of the neck in a patient about to undergo surgery for goitre? Which views are commonly requested?**
   Ans: To check for tracheal deviation or compression which is usually symptomatic but a warning sign that respiratory obstruction might develop postoperative. AP lateral and thoracic inlet views are usually requested. A multinodular goiter may show calcification.
6. **Which are the specific early complications of thyroidectomy?**
   Ans: 1st early reactionary hemorrhage, recurrent laryngeal nerve palsy or temporary paresis. Thyroid crisis.
   2nd–3rd day: Hypocalcemia due to parathyroid damage. Presents as circumoral tingling, Chvostek's and Trousseau's signs positive.
   4th day: Wound infection.
7. **Patient five hours after thyroidectomy is distressed, frightened, and breathless with a swollen neck and tachycardia. What is the treatment?**
   Ans: The diagnosis is either tracheal compression due to reactionary hemorrhage or acute thyroid crisis. Sit the patient up: start 100% oxygen by mask: give a small amount of sedation, e.g. diazepam 5 mg i.v. if the pulse rate is below 150/min. Thyroid crisis looks like thyrotoxicosis, i.e. tachycardia, restlessness, pyrexia, tremor. It responds to more Diazepam+Propranolol i.v. Tracheal compression, breathlessness, stridor, cyanosis, cut the stitches and clips and the deep vertical layer of stitches in the strap muscles, evaluate the clot and place a light *in situ*. If the stridor continues you need an anesthetist, and the patient will need to go back to theatre anyway.
8. **What mnemonic summaries the presentation of hypercalcaemia?**
   Ans: Stones, bones and abdominal groans hypocalcemia alone, patients who are significantly symptomatic and unable to take oral medications should be taken with sufficient intravenous calcium gluconate solution to control symptoms. Serum calcium levels should be obtained every 12 hours. Hypocalcemia persisting after the first few postoperative days should initially be treated with oral calcium alone to avoid the problems of initiating and weaning from vitamin D therapy. Overt hypocalcaemia persisting for more than 10 to 14 days postoperatively is best treated with a combination of oral calcium and a vitamin D preparation. This vitamin D preparation should contain the one alpha-hydroxyl functionally group because other forms of vitamin D are not readily hydroxylated in this position to form 1,25-dihydroxy vitamin D in stated of diminished PTH.
9. **How does recurrent laryngeal nerve injury occur?**
   Ans: Recurrent laryngeal nerve injury occurs from excessive trauma to the nerve during explosure, inclusion of the nerve in a ligature, or inadvertent sectioning of the nerve. The damage may be unilateral or bilateral and temporary or permanent.

10. **What are physical and laryngoscopic findings of unilateral recurrent laryngeal nerve injury?**
Ans: On physical examination, paralysis of one vocal cord (caused by nerve injury) results in a huskiness of the voice with verifying degrees of hoarseness. On laryngoscopic examination the vocal cord will be found assuming a median or paramedian position because of abductor laryngeal paralysis. In the presence of hoarness unassociated with laryngoscopic abnormalities, the most likely cause is vocal cord edema from intubation; this is usually adequately treated with humidification of inspired air.

11. **What treatment is required in unilateral injury?**
Ans: In unilateral injury, cord paralysis results in narrowing of the glottis aperture, which is not sufficient to cause airway obstruction unless concurrent glottis edema is present. If the injury is related to dissection and the nerve is intact, function usually returns within 3 to 6 months. Typically, asymptomatic unilateral cord paralysis does not require treatment.

12. **What is the role for medical therapy in primary hyperparathyroidism?**
Ans: Although surgery is the mainstay of treatment in primarily hyperparathyroidism, medical therapy is used in cases life-threatening hypercalcemia and in patients who have unacceptable surgical risks.

13. **What is the presentation of acute primarily hyperparathyroidism (hyperparathyroid crisis)?**
Ans: Hyperparathyroidism seldom presents as acute life-threatening hypercalcemia, and typically with serum calcium levels >14.0 mg/dl and central nervous system disorders (confusion, disorientation, or coma), gastrointestinal problems (anorexia, nausea, or weight loss), or neuromuscular dysfunction (fatigue or muscle weakness). The precipitating cause is usually volume depletion stress. Two-thirds of these patients will have diagnostic features of hyperparathyroidism (past history of hypercalcemia, presence of nephrolithiasis or nephrocalcinosis, or radiographically demonstrated bone disease.

14. **What is the treatment of this disorder?**
Ans: Emergency treatment consists of volume depletion with intravenous saline followed by furosemide to promote a sodium (and consequent calcium) diuresis. Mithramcycin, through its inhibition of osteoclastic activity; is often effective in preventing further accelerated bone resorption. Potassium and magnesium administration is important to replace the large losses of these ions.

15. **List the classic symptoms of hyperthyroidism?**
Ans: Feeling, hot, insensitivity to cold weight loss, tremor, diarrhoea, menstrual upset–usually oligomenorrhage. Mental agitation/anxiety. Eye changes–protuberance, double vision, discomfort, warm sweaty hands.

16. **What is the differences diagnosis of a diffuse from thyroid swelling in a woman of 35?**
Ans:
(i) Hashimoto's disease–gland is rubbery
(ii) Anaplastic carcinoma–gland is woody hard
(iii) Medullary carcinoma–rare (C cells)
(iv) Graves' disease–diffusely enlarged thyroid is accompanied by gross thyrotoxicosis.

17. **How does their position allow you to distinguish between thyroglossal cyst, thyroglossal fistula, branchial cyst, branchial fistula and pharyngeal pouch?**
Ans: Thyroglossal cyst: Always in midline. Usually between hyoid bone and thyroid cartilage. Protrusion of tongue makes cyst move. Thyroglossal fistula: Midline tract associated with the above. Branchial cyst: Lies near angle of jaw in upper third of neck

partly behind sternomastoid. Branchial fistula; cyst: Lies on anterior border of sternomastoid and may communicate with branchial cyst. Pharyngeal pouch: Lies in midline third of neck, deep in posterior triangle. Can be emptied into pharynx by firm pressure.

18. How may a goiter cause acute respiratory obstruction?

Ans: Spontaneous haemorrhage (into a depression nodule) within the thyroid, and this may be retrosternal.

19. What are the main causes of postoperative respiratory obstruction after thyroidectomy?

Ans: Damaged recurrent laryngeal nerve(s) (cord adduct). Tracheal collapse–tracheomalacia. Postoperative haematoma (leading to venous congestion and laryngeal edema).

20. When you examine a patient with a goiter, what are the main clinical features that you must establish that will effect how you further investigate and treat the patient?

Ans: Goitre: Multinodular or single lump. Palpable local lymph nodes. Recurrent laryngeal nerve paresis.

Thyroid status hypo/hyper/euthyroid

21. List the clinical features of Cushing's syndrome, briefly

Ans: Cushingoid facies: Moon face, acne, striae, bruising, etc. Buffalo neck hump: weight gain, muscle wasting and weakness, hypertension, amenorrhoea, susceptibility to infections, and many more.

22. Once you have established a diagnosis of Cushing's syndrome you need to establish its causes. List four different sources for the excess glucocorticoids

Ans:

(i) Iatrogenic (Gk iater = physician) steroid treatment, e.g. prednisolone. This made Cushing's syndrome a common condition.
(ii) Overproduction by the adrenal(s): Hyperplasia and tumour
(iii) Excess pituitary ACTH: Pituitary tumour
(iv) Ectopic ACTH production: Carcinoma or adenoma or bronchus is the commonest.

23. Hormone secreting tumours of the pancreas may give rise to three types of endocrine disorder. Name these

Ans:

(i) Hypoglycaemic attacks from insulinoma
(ii) Intractable peptic ulceration from gastrinoma
(iii) Waterly diarrhoea from VIP oma.

24. What are the two main types of hyperthyroidism?

Ans: Grave's disease (diffuse hyperplasia) and Plummer's disease (toxic nodule).

25. What is the cause of hyperthyroidism?

Ans: Immunoglobulin, stimulating, thyroid-stimulating hormone (TSH), causes thyroid cells to release excess thyroxin (Graves' disease). Hyperplastic cell release excess thyroxin (Plummer's disease).

26. What is the chief clinical differences between solitary and multiple thyroid nodules?

Ans: Multiple thyroid nodules are considered benign unless some finding (laryngeal nerve palsy, firmness, enlarged nodes, rapid growth) suggests malignancy. Solitary thyroid nodules are considered malignant until proved benign. A previous history of irradiation of any of the above findings strongly suggests malignancy.

27. Does a "cold" nodule on thyroid scintiscan indicate malignancy?
Ans: All cysts and many benign adenomas show up as cold nodules. A few thyroid cancers to shrink malignant ones. Soft nodules, especially those appearing during pregnancy, will often regress on suppression. Aspiration biopsy cytology is, of course, more accurate in differentiating benign from malignant nodules.

28. Should solitary thyroid nodules be suppressed with thyroxin for 3–6 months to indicate whether it is benign or malignant?
Ans: Suppression often fails to shrink benign nodules, and in some cases it has been reported to shrink malignant ones. Soft nodules, especially those appearing during pregnancy, will often regress on suppression. Aspiration biopsy cytology is, of course, more accurate in differentiating benign from malignant nodules.

29. What is the most common cancer diagnosed by aspiration biopsy cytology?
Ans: Papillary cancer (ground-glass nuclei and psammoma bodies).

30. What malignancy is the best reliably diagnosed by aspiration biopsy cytology?
Ans: Papillary cancer (Note: This is why most follicular nodules are excised).

31. What are the main types of solitary thyroid nodules?
Ans: Nodular goiter with one

		Cancer 20%	
Dominant nodule	50%	thyroiditis	5%
Adenoma	20%	cysts	5%

32. What is management of solitary thyroid nodules?
Ans: Perform lobectomy of side of nodule and thyroid supplements.

33. What is common types of thyroiditis?
Ans: Lymphocytic hashmotos thyroiditis and diffuse goiter.

34. What are the cause of hypercalcemia?
Ans: Bone metasis, hyperparathyroidism and thiazide diuretics.

35. What are symptoms of hyper parathyroidism?
Ans: Bones–pain, fractures
Stones–renal stones
Abdominal–pancreatitis, peptic ulcers and listlessness.

36. What are tests to diagnosis hyperparathyroidism?
Ans: Serum calcium 3 times normals
Elevated parathormone
Elevated alkaline phosphatase
Decreased phosphatase

37. Describe parathyroid embryology?
Ans: Upper pair branchial arch IV
Lower pair from branchial arch III

38. What is pathology OP primary hyperparathyroidism?
Ans: Single adenoma 85%
Diffuse hyperplasia 11%
Double adenoma 3%
Cancer <1%

39. What are localizing tests?
Ans: Thallium technetium scan localize parathyroid tissue 70%, ultrasound.

40. What is treatment?
Ans: For calcium <11 observe for 12 months for calcium more than 11 MG/DL exploration is done.

41. What are complication of surgery for parathyroid?
Ans. Chvostek sign–tapping facial nerve
Elicits spasm of facial muscles
Trousseau–occluding brachial artery for 3 minutes includes carpal spasms.

Flow Chart: Thyrotoxicosis

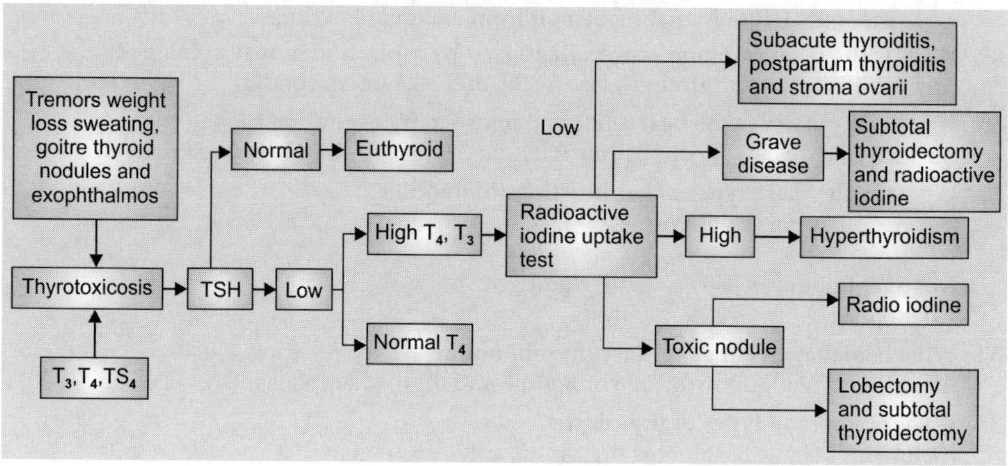

Flow Chart: Goitre

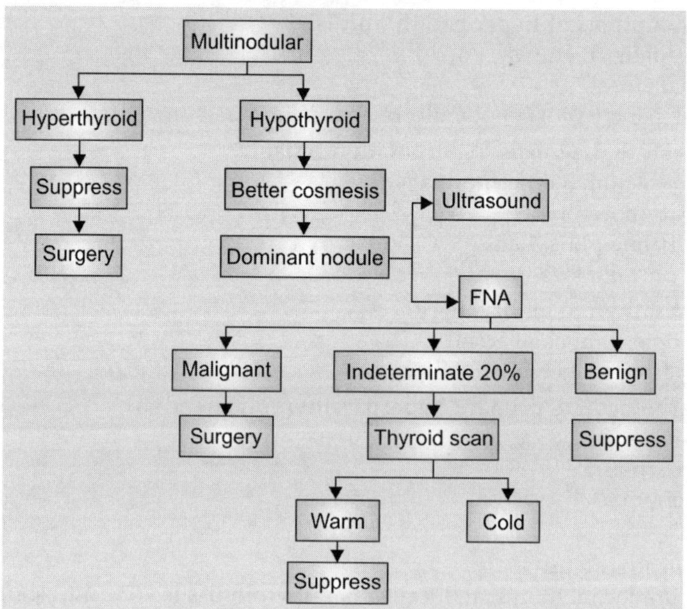

Flow Chart: Thyroid carcinoma

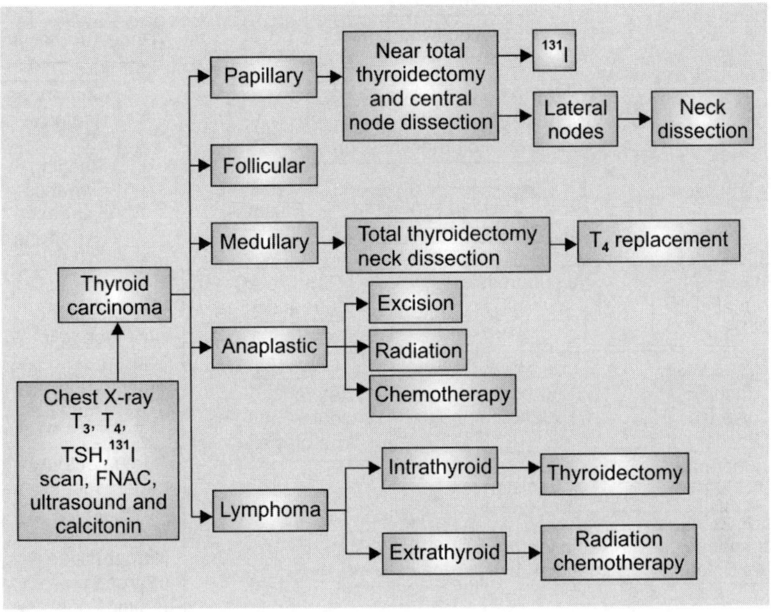

Flow Chart: Hyperparathyroidism

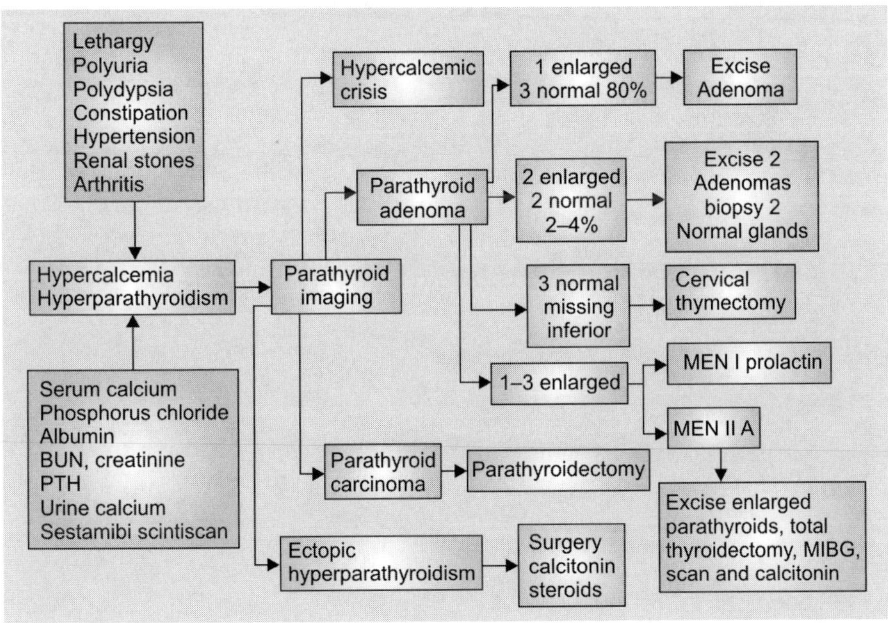

Flow Chart: Adrenal tumour

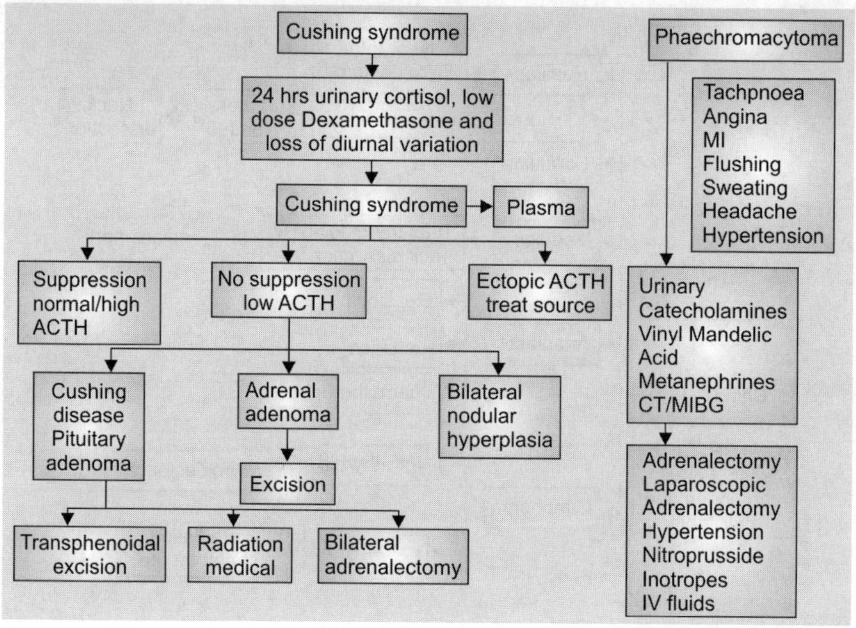

11

Esophagus

ANATOMIC POINTS OF INTEREST

A. Fibromuscular tube extending from cricopharyngeal sphincter to cardia of stomach below diaphragm.
B. Two layers striated muscle upper one-third, smooth muscle lower two-thirds. Fibromuscular tube 25 cm extending from cricopharyngeal sphincter to cardia of stomach. 2 cm below diaphragm with 3 constrictions, 15 cm–cricopharyngeal, 25 cm–aortic, 40 cm–diaphragm.
C. Muscle with no serosa
D. Squamous epithelium–columnar epithelium
E. No anatomic lower esophageal sphincter (LES)–physiologic only, relying on unique.
F. Blood pressure from aortic via direct and anastomosing branches.
G. Lies in posterior mediastinum in chest–right side of midline, upper two-thirds, left side of midline on lower one-third.
H. Parasympathetic nerves supply mediated by vagus through extrinsic and intrinsic plexus. Intrinsic plexus has no Meissner's network which is present elsewhere in alimentary canal and only Auerbach plexus is present.

PHYSIOLOGY

A. General
   1. Peristaltic wave–voluntary up high, then involuntary propagation.
   2. LES relaxes to accept food, then returns to normal resting pressure (15–25 cm H_2O above pressure in stomach).
   3. Transfer food from mouth to stomach in coordinated manner. Failure to relax on swallowing may predispose to development of pharyngeal pouch (pulsion diverticulum).
B. Assessment
   1. Esophageal manometry diagnose esophageal motility disorders: Small catheter with pressure transducers at 5 cm intervals which track pressure wave through swallowing mechanisms. Recording are made by passing multilumen catheter with 3–8 recording orifices at different levels. Recording are taken at intervals of 1 cm to measure length, pressure of lower oesophageal sphincter.
   2. pH monitoring to evaluate reflux esophagitis, pH probe is passed at distal oesophagus 5 cm above lower oesophageal sphincter. Probe is connected to

miniature digital recorder worn as belt. 24 hr pH recording is analysed. In healthy adults pH < does not exceed 4% in 24 hours.

3. Barium swallow
4. Oesophagoscopy

PATHOLOGY

A. Motility disorders
   1. Cricopharyngeal muscle dysfunction–Zenker diverticula (post-midline)-pulsion type
      a. Symptoms of regurgitation, putrid breath odor
      b. Treated with excision of redundant mucosa and myotomy
      c. Surgery with linear stapler with common in septum.
   2. Epiphrenic diverticula–often do not need treatment.
   3. Achalasia–inability to relax lower oesophageal sphincter–dilated esophagus–Bird's break appearance–more dysphagia with liquid than solids. Rx with balloon dilatation or Heller myotomy. Loss of ganglion cells in myenteric (Auerbach's plexus). Laparoscopic Heller's myotomy. Loss of ganglion cells in myenteric (Auerbach's plexus). Laparoscopic Heller's myotomy is treatment of choice.
   4. 'Nutcracker' esophagus–increased motility–chest pain, Rx NTG, nifedipine. Manometry shows mean amplitude >180 mm Hg (normal 30–120 mm Hg).
   5. Presbyesophagus–tertiary contraction.
   6. Scleroderma–poor or no motility–difficulty swallowing, weight loss.

B. WEBS–Plummer Vinson, (Patersonbrown-Kelly) syndrome. Thin web above cricopharyngeal sphincter causes glossitis dysphagia and anaemia. Treatment is stretching or rupturing by endoscopy. Kremer Schatzi at upper border of gastroesophageal junction above hiatus hernia causes dysphagia. Treatment is dilatation.

C. Oesophageal rupture may be spontaneous or iatrogenic (Boerhaave syndrome) causes chest pain, dysphagia. Diagnosis is by water soluble contrast study. Treatment is surgical repair.

D. Barret's oesophagus is circumferential columnar lined oesophagus for more than 3 cm and endoscopic appearance is salmon pink and treatment is PPI and esophagectomy if invasive carcinoma is found.

E. Oesophageal stricture could be peptic, Barrett's corrective. Treatment is dilation and Stent placement. Perforation requires oesophagectomy.

F. Reflux esophagitis (GERD).
   1. Often associated with sliding hiatus hernias (Type 1).
   2. Prevalence is 5% and symptoms are heartburn, epigastric and retrosternal pain, regurgitation related to meals, lying down and straining.
   3. There is normal oesophageal motility, LOS intrinsic pressure, positive pressure on intra-abdominal oesophageal motility and resting pressure of LOS.

4. 24 hours ambulatory pH and stationary manometry with ten wet swallows to determine oesophageal motility and resting pressure of LOS.
5. Management is to stop smoking, reduce alcohol, loose weight, raise head end bed, avoid precipitating foods and acids, eating <3 hours before bed, H_2 blockers, proton pump inhibitors, pro-kinetic drugs. Surgical repair are Nissen's fundoplication and Toupet fundoplication. Laparoscopic Nissen's fundoplication is becoming gold standards for GERD. It involves posterior crural repair, division of short gastric vessels, and 360 wrap around distal oesophagus, 85% have symptomatic relief.

Hiatus Hernia

Protrusion of viscus through oesophageal hiatus. Distinction by endoscopy and barium swallow/meal.

Classification

1. Paraoesophageal hernia or rolling (10%): The competent oesophagogastric junction (OGJ) may lie above the diaphragm, but the apex of the hernia is formed by a pouch of stomach which herniates alongside the lower oesophagus.
2. Sliding hernia (80%): Where an incompetent oesophagogastric junction forms the apex of the hernia and lies above diaphragm complications are of reflux oesophagitis stricture and oesophageal shortening are seen.
3. Combined (10%).

THEORIES OF AETIOLOGY

1. Primarily an anatomical abnormality in the obese middle aged where weak ligaments and muscles fail to anchor the OGJ in its infradiaphragmatic position. The stomach is then displaced into the posterior mediastinum.
2. The result of excessive traction by esophageal longitudinal muscle hauling the oesophagogastric junction into the posterior mediastinum. The functional abnormality may be caused by abnormal neuromuscular coordination or by gastrointestinal hormonal imbalance, factors which may eventually correlate with the high incidence of obesity, cholelithiasis, gastric hypermobility and hypersection in these patients.

Factors Contributing to OGJ Competence

1. A length of intra-abdominal oesophagus which implies obliquely into the stomach forming an acute with the fundus.
2. The presence of an intrinsic lower oesophagus sphincter.
3. A compressed abdominal oesophagus, the result of its lumen being at intrathoracic (negative) pressure lying in the positive pressure of the abdomen.
4. The support given to the abdominal oesophagus by the right crus of diaphragm.

Conservative for Surgery

85% of symptomatic patients can be altered successfully.

1. Weight loss: Sleep propped upright.
2. No food or drink after early evening.
3. Preparations to protect oesophageal mucosa, e.g. antacids, silicones and alginates.

Indications for Surgery

1. Failure to respond to conservative management
2. Peptic strictures
3. Oesophageal ulceration discrete enough to see on barium swallow
4. Respiratory complications from the reflux of oesophageal contents into the trachea. Productive cough, lung abscess, or even empyema can occur
5. Significant anaemia and hemorrhage
6. A huge hiatus hernia causing postprandial cardiorespiratory distress
7. During laparotomy for concomitant conditions, (e.g. duodenal ulceration, cholelithiasis).

Surgical Relief of Symptoms

All the surgical procedures described are designed to achieve one or more of the following objectives:

1. Closure of hiatus by apposition of the two limbs of right crus
2. Anchoring of the OGJ in its sub-diaphragmatic position
   i. By suturing the oesophagus to the opposed right crus
   ii. By gastropexy
3. Construction of an acute angle between the abdominal oesophagus and the gastric fundus by:
   i. Suturing the fundus to oesophagus
   ii. Suturing the fundus to the under surface of the left diaphragm
   iii. Wrapping the fundus around the suturing it to the abdominal oesophagus (Nissen fundoplication)
4. Weakening of the oesophageal longitudinal muscle by:
   i. Circumference oesophageal myotomy
   ii. Multiple, short sector myotomies
5. Adequate gastric drainage if there is an element of duodenal stenosis
6. A lowering of any gastric hypersecretion by vagotomy.

Specific Surgical Procedures

1. Fundoplication
   i. Reduction of hernia at laparotomy.
   ii. A wide bore stomach tube is passed into the oesophagus to prevent too a closure of right crus.

iii. The margins of the right crus are defined and approximated behind the oesophagus.
iv. Mobilisation of the proximal stomach by division of gastrosplenic omentum.
v. The mobilized fundus is wrapped around and sutured in front of the abdominal.
vi. Vagotomy, pyloroplasty can be added.

2. Belsey operation
   i. Thoractomy through bed of 7th or 8th rib.
   ii. The acute angle of entry of the oesophagus into the stomach, and a length of intra-abdominal oesophageal is produced by a series of mattress sutures which pass from the oesophagus (a few cm above oesophagogastric junction); to the fundus (an equal distance from oesophagogastric junction) to the diaphragm from below upwards; (2 cm from the hernia ring) then through the diaphragm to pick up fundus and oesophagus again.
   iii. The right crus is then approximated behind the oesophagus.
3. Collis operation
   i. Left thoracoabdominal approach.
   ii. Approximation of right crus in front of oesophagus.
   iii. The fundus of the stomach is sutured to the under surface of left dome of diaphragm to maintain an acute angle between the abdominal oseophagus and stomach.
4. Gastropexy
   i. Anterior gastropexy: Fixation of anterior surface of stomach (adjacent to lesser curve) to the linea alba.
   ii. Hill posterior gastropexy: Fixation of lesser curve (and posterior phreno-oesophageal ligament) to median arcuate ligament.

Carcinoma of Oesophagus

Six fold increased in last 25 years with male female incidence is 5:1. Associated with tobacco/ETOH abuse, diet, vitamin deficiency, Barret's oesophagus and Plummer Vinson syndrome and caustic burns.

Oesophageal Subdivision

Squamous cell carcinoma 50% upper and middle third.

Adenocarcinoma 50% lower 1/3, spread could be extension to mediastinal pleura, pericardium, lymphathetic and blood borne to lung and liver.

Spread of Oesophageal Carcinoma

1. Direct spread
   i. Submucosal spread
   ii. Longitudinal or circumferential
   iii. Transmural

2. Lymphatic spread
   i. Intramural lymphatic permeation and embolisation. Clearance of 6 cm of 'normal' oesophagus is required. Access to a sufficient length of 'normal' oesophagus dictates the surgical approach and forms the rational basis for total oesophagectomy.
   ii. Upper third : Cervical lymph nodes
   Middle third : Hilar and subcarinal nodes, or to celiac nodes
   Lower third : Celiac nodes
3. Blood borne spread to liver, bone, skin.

Clinical Features

Dysphagia, weight loss, bleeding, reflux symptoms, odynophagia and RLN palsy.

Diagnosis

Barium swallow shows shouldered strictures and rat tail appearance. Biopsy, Brush cytology, X-ray chest, endolumial ultrasound, bronchoscopy, laparoscopy, laparoscopic ultrasound and mediastinoscopy.

Classification

TNM
T_{IS} Carcinoma *in situ*
T_1 Invading lamina/submucosa
T Invading muscularis propria
T_3 Invading adventitia
T_4 Invasion of adjacent structures
N_0 No nodal spread
N_1 Regional lymph nodes
N_2 Distant metasis.

Surgical to Carcinoma Lower Third Oesophagus

1. Tumors below the diaphragm (unless there is peritoneal or abdominal visceral spread) can be excised radically through a left thoracoabdominal approach together with stomach, spleen, tail of pancreas, omentum, the regional lymphathetic field and restoring continuously by oesophagojejunal anastomosis en-Roux, or esophagogastrostomy.
2. Trans-hiatal oesophagectomy: Abdominal and left neck incision suitable for anastomosis in neck for distal third tumours.
3. Carcinoma above the diaphragm should be excised by the Lewis-Tanner operation (the two stages procedure). Access to sufficient length of 'normal' oesophagus is not possible through a left throacoabdominal approach. The stomach is mobilized on the right gastric and gastroepiploic arteries at laparotomy, and Kocher procedure and pyloromyotomy are performed. Through a right thoracotomy, the tumour and lower oesophagus are

mobilized and the stomach is drawn into the chest. The tumour with adequate clearance of 'normal' oesophagus and the proximal stomach are resected and continuity is restored by oesophagogastric anastomosis.

Surgical to Carcinoma Middle Third Oesophagus

1. For carcinoma in the lower half of the middle third of oesophagus, the Lewis-Tanner operation can be performed.
2. When a carcinoma of the upper half of the middle third is removed by the two-stage procedure then to allow adequate clearance above the tumour, the oesophagogastric anastomosis will have to be performed high in the superior mediastinum. The dangers of such a difficult anastomosis can be reduced by a three stage total oesophagectomy. The third stage involves the mobilization of the cervical oesophagus through a right supraclavicular incision; the delivery of the oesophagus into the neck wound; oesophagectomy with closure of the oesophagogastric junction; and restoration of continuity by anastomosing the cervical oesophagus with gastric fundus.

Treatment of Carcinoma of Upper Third Oesophagus

1. The three stages total oesophagectomy. McKeown three stage oesophagectomy
2. Radiotherapy

The Place of Radiotherapy in Carcinoma of Oesophagus

1. It has been claimed that megavoltage irradiation to squamous carcinoma of oesophagus offers a better 5-year survival than surgery. One of the reasons for this was the absence of treatment morbidity following irradiation. However, the surgical series used for comparison with radiotherapy was collected between 1948 and 1963, since when improvement in techniques will have improved operative mortality. Adenocarcinoma of oesophagus (10% of total) arising from oesophageal mucous glands is radioresistant.
2. Postoperative radiotherapy to known residual tumour may improve the surgical rate. However, if the stoma lies within the field of irradiation, stomal necrosis may occur. In the three stages total oesophagectomy, the stoma is outside the field of irradication, allowing safe irradication of hilar and carinal nodes.

Treatment of Unresectable Carcinoma of Oesophagus

About 50% of carcinoma of middle third of oesophagus are unresectable.

QUESTIONS AND ANSWERS

1. **What is the most commonly cause of portal hypertension in the US in adults in children?**
   Ans: Cirrhosis of the liver, most frequently caused by chronic alcoholism, is the most common use of portal hypertension in Western countries. Alcoholic cirrhosis causes obstruction of portal venous blood flow on the hepatic vein, side of the sinusoid (postsinusoidal). Laennee's cirrhosis account for 85% of cases of portal hypertension in

the US extrahepatic portal venous occlusion is the second most common cause of portal hypertension and is the most common cause of portal hypertension in children. This is the most commonly a consequence of cavernous malformation of the portal vein.

2. **Which vein join to form the portal vein?**
   Ans: The portal vein 8–9 cm in length and is formed by the confluence of the splenic and superior mesenteric veins. The portal vein lies dorsal and medial to the common bile duct and hepatic artery in the hepatoduodenal ligament. There are no valves in the portal circulation.
3. **The most likely diagonosis based on the history in the patient is**
   A. Cancer of the esophagus
   B. Achalasia (cardiospasm)
   C. Peptic esophagitis with secondary strictures
   D. All of these
   Ans: (a) A patient with progressive dysphagia and weight loss almost always has a mechanical obstruction of his esophagus. Whether it is due to a malignant or a benign condition is determined by esophagoscopy and biopsy. Cancer of the oesophagus produces an insidious, but progressive dysphagia which will ultimately progress to complete obstruction. Duration of syndromes prior to diagonosis is variable, but average 4 and 6 months.
4. **What risks or predisposing factors are linked with an increased incidence of cancer of the esophagus?**
   A. Excessive smoking
   B. Achalasia (Cardiospasm)
   C. Excessive alcohol consumption
   D. Corrosive lye strictures of the oesophagus
   E. All of these
5. **The most common area of the esophagus involved by cancer is**
   A. Cervical esophagus
   B. Upper thoracic esophagus
   C. Lower thoracic esophagus
   D. Esophagogastric junction
   Ans: (d) Esophagogastric junction is most frequently involved. However, 50% of all cancers occurring at the esophagogastric junction are adenocarcinomas of gastric origin and should properly be classified as stomach cancer rather than esophageal.
6. **What is the role of radiotherapy in the treatment of oesophageal cancer?**
   Ans: Radiation therapy may be used to cure esophageal cancer or palliate symptoms. If palliative , a dosage in the range of 20 to 30 Gy (2000 to 3000 rad) over a 2-week period may provide temporary alleviation of such distributing symptoms as pain, hemorrhage, and dysphagia with relatively little morbidity. Radical treatment for curve necessitates a dosage of 50 to 60 Gy delivered over a period of 4 or more weeks. This forms of treatment is not without risk, for such complications include tracheoesophageal fistula, radiation myelitis, hemorrhage and constrictive pericarditis. Preoperatives radiation in lesser doses of 20 to 50 Gy appears to improve the respectability rate modestly without affecting survival.
7. **Is chemotherapy effective treatment?**
   Ans: Chemotherapy alone has had little demonstrate effect in palliating patients with squamous cell carcinoma of the esophagus. Because of the belief that this disease is often

systemic at the time of diagnosis, combined modality treatment using chemotherapy, radiation therapy, and resection in a staged regimen has gained popularity.

8. **If a patient is not a candidate for a curative resection, how can dysphagia be palliated?**

Ans: Esophagectomy can produce unobstructed swallowing in more than 90% of patients throughout their subsequently survival, but should be performed only if the risks are minimal and at least one year survival is reasonable. Intubation of the esophagus with a prosthetic tube such as the Celestin tube has been used for many years to allow patients to swallow. Recently, endoscopic dilatation and laser treatment have been used to reestablish esophageal continuity through malignant obstruction. Radiations therapy relieves dysphagia partially or completely is almost 80% of patients, although the effect is temporary.

9. **What is Barrett's esophagus?**

Ans: Barett's esophagus is a columnar-lined esophagus resulting from glandular mucosa replacing the normal squamous cell mucosa. Chronic gastroesophageal reflux is the cause.

10. **What is the relationships between Barrett's esophagus and adenocarcinoma of the esophagus?**

Ans: Fifty nine to 86% of adenocarcinomas of the esophagus arise in a Barrett's esophagus. The percentages of patient with Barrett's esophagus who subsequently develop adenocarcinoma ranges from 0 to 46.5 %. Little is known about the factors responsible for the malignant degeneration of this tissue. In theory, chronic gastroesophageal reflux leads to esophagitis, then hyperplasia, dysplasia, carcinoma in situ, and, finally invasive carcinoma.

11. **What is portal hypertension?**

Ans: Portal hypertension is an elevation in pressure of the portal venous circulation. Normal portal venous pressure ranges from 7–10 mm Hg, whereas average portal pressure in portal hypertension is 20 mm Hg with a range of 15–60 mm Hg.

12. **What are the causes of portal hypertension?**

Ans: Portal hypertension may be caused by increased resistance to portal blood flow or increased portal blood flow. Increased resistance to flow is divided into three main categories (1) prehepatic (portal vein thrombosis, extrinsic compression [tumours]; (2) hepatic (cirrhosis, congenital hepatic, fibrosis, schistosomiasis); and (3) post-hepatic (Budd-Chiari syndrome, constrictive pericarditis). Increased portal blood flow may be caused by arterial-portal venous fistulas or increased splenic flow, as seen in various forms of splenomegaly.

13. **What is anatomy of esophagus?**

Ans: Esophagus begins at C6 below cricoids cartilage. Length of esophagus is 23–30 cm. It extends till gastroesophageal junction. Inferior thyroid artery supplies cervical portion (thoracic by branches for aorta and esophageal branches of bronchial arteries). Lymphatic system is composed of two lymphatic plexus in mucosa, submucosa which communicates with network of lymphatic vessels.

14. **What is surgical treatment of esophageal cancer?**

Ans: Esophagectomy with esophagogastrostomy is preferred treatment of esophageal cancer. The two most commonly performed procedure are ivor-lewis esophagectomy through abdominal and cervical incisions. Pyloromyotomy is done in cases where colonic interposition is to be constructed to provide conduit to stomach left colon is used.

Flow Chart: Benign stricture

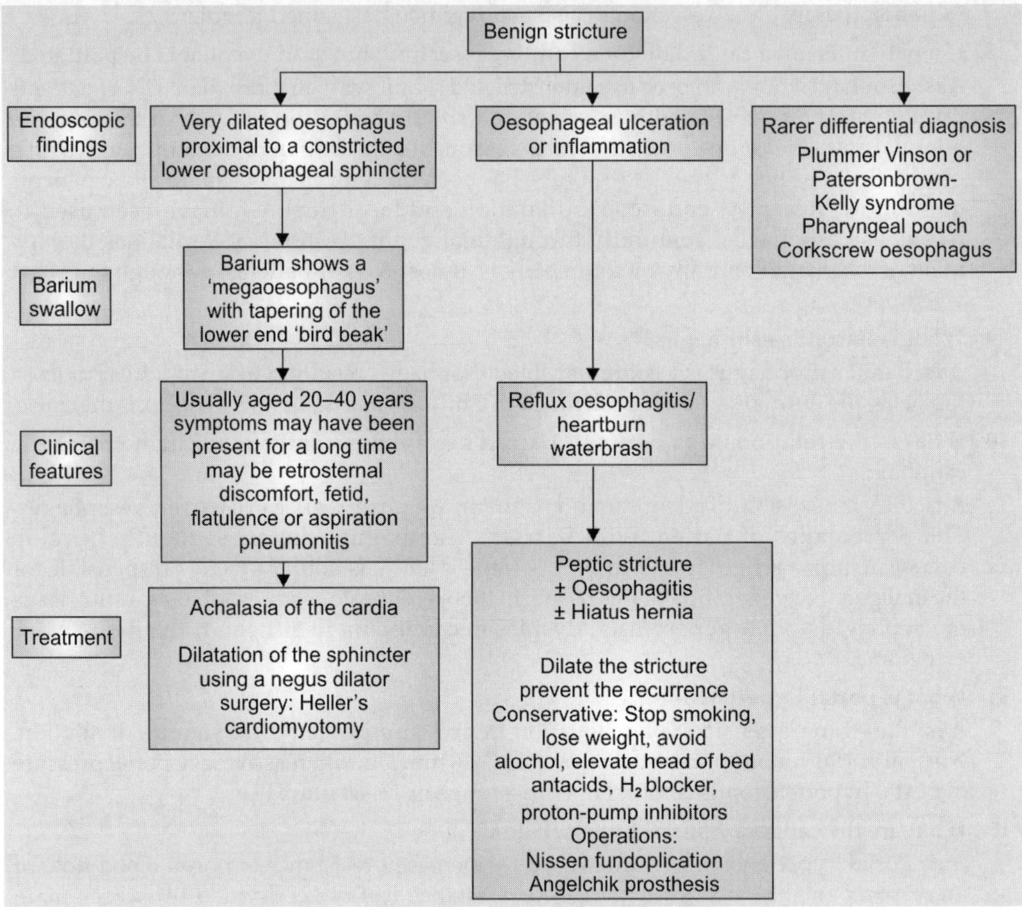

Flow Chart: Achalasia

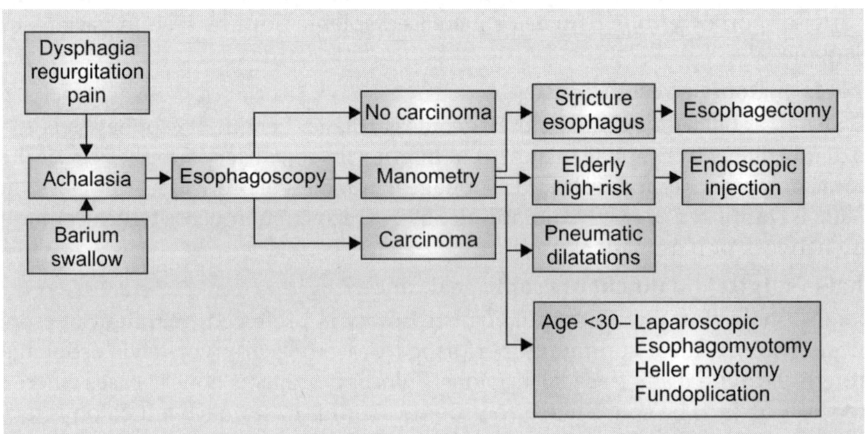

Flow Chart: Esophagus stricture

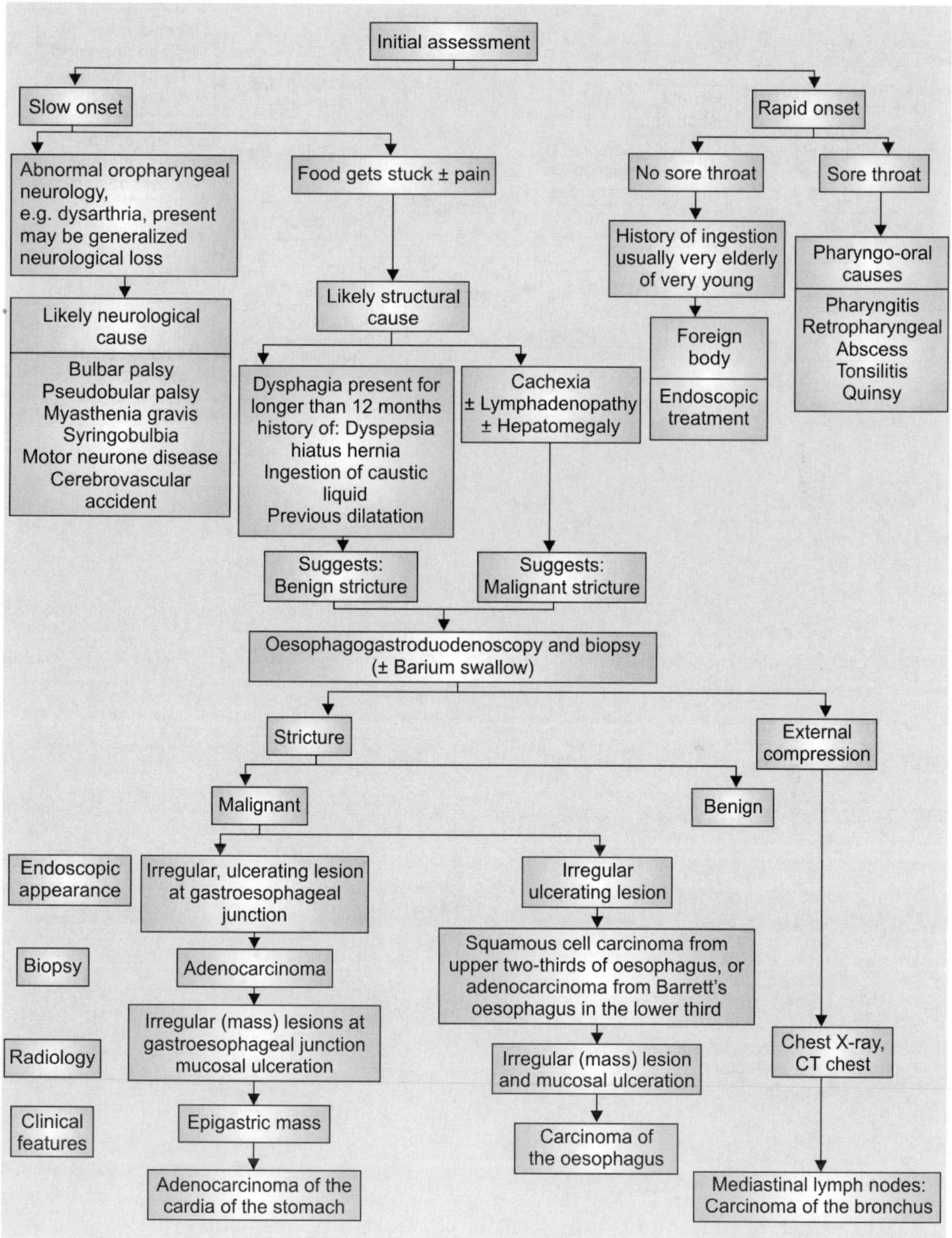

Flow Chart: Carcinoma esophagus

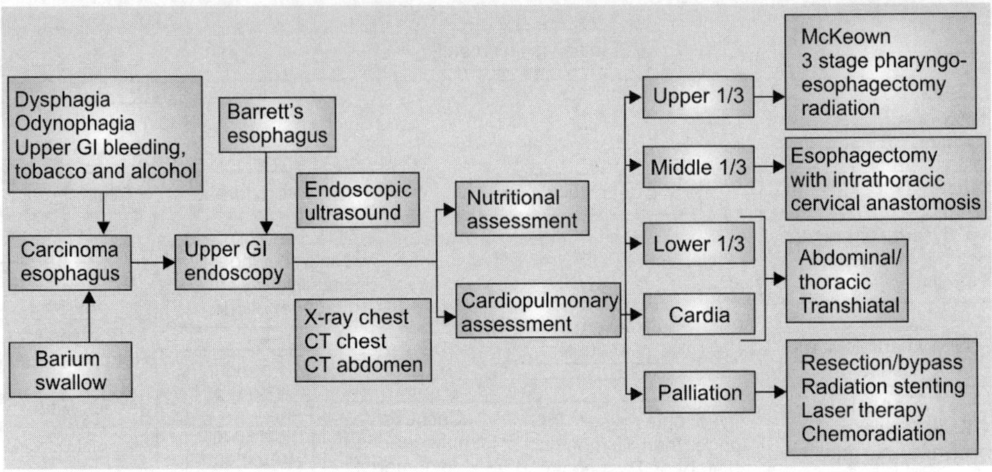

12

Stomach

ANATOMY

- Stomach has two surface (anterior and posterior), two curvatures (greater and lesser) and two orifices (cardia and pylorous).
- Gastrooesophageal junction is known as cardia and 2.5 cm left of midline at level of T_{10}. Distal 1/5 of stomach is comprising of pyloric antrum, and sphincter. Pyloroduodenal junction is identified by vein of Mayo is to right of midline of level L_1. Pyloric sphincter comprises of outer longitudinal and inner vascular muscle layer. Cardiac sphincter has rosette like mucosal folds and acute angle of lower esophagus into stomach acts as a value like effects.
- Blood supply consists of:
  1. Arterial supply consisting of left gastric artery from celiac axis, right artery from hepatic artery, right gastroepiploic artery from gastroduodenal branch of hepatic artery, left gastroepiploic artery from splenic artery and short gastric from splenic artery.
  2. Sympathetic fibre (Vasomotor) accompanied by afferent pain fibre run with various arterial branches to stomach. Parasympathetic supply is from vagus which controls motility and secretion.
  3. Lymph drains parallel to greater curvature of stomach and 2/3 down the anterior surface along left gastric artery. From zone above and right lymph bases to left and right gastric along left gastric artery. From upper left quadrant it flows to pancreaticosplenic nodes rest of greater curvatures it drain into subpyloric nodes. Pyloric region drain into hepatic and left gastric nodes. Lymph from stomach eventually reaches coeliac nodes through subgroups.

PHYSIOLOGY

- Acts as a reservoir, produces chyme and regulate gastric emptying.
- Produce gastric juice which is water, HCl, electrolytes, H^+ ions, Na^+ 40 mm; K 10 mm, Cl 150 mm pepsin, mucus, intrinsic factor gastric lipase, blood group of ABO system (columnar cells of gastric mucosa and mucus neck cells).
- Pepsin is secreted by inactive precursor pepsinogen/by peptic cell of gastric gland. Intrinsic factor by glycol protein by parietal cells.

Specific tests for gastric cancer include tumour markers CEA (which is elevated in 1/3 gastric tumors). Combining CEA, CA 19-9, other tests include endoscopy, endoscopic ultrasound and CT scan and laparoscopy and PET.

Cephalic phase is induced by thought smell which stimulates hypothalamus–dorsal motor nucleus of vagus. Taste fibre from oral receptors along nucleus of trackus solataris–dorsal vagal nucleus.

Gastric phase is by distension of fundus and body of stomach leads to stimulation of stretch receptor–stimulates receptors of myenteric plexus causing acid secretion. Intestinal phase is result of gastric release from cells in duodenal mucosa. Gastric–elderly lesser air valve.

DIAGNOSTIC TOOLS

- Radiography–barium swallow, upper gastrointestinal (UGI) series–easy, relatively cheap, 80–90% sensitivity/specificity.
- Endoscopy–flexible "EGD" esophagogastroduodenoscopy–very safe/accurate–can be biopsied
- Acid analysis
  1. Basal acid output
  2. Maximum output–stimulated by histamine or pentagastrin and inhibited by secreting
  3. Gastric emptying studies include insulin tests, 24 hrs intragastric pH monitoring and bile reflux gastropathy.

PEPTIC ULCER

- Associated with light basal acid output, type A personality, blood group A and *H. pylori* infections which is worlds most common bacterial infections (75%).
- Clinical features OGD, upper GI endoscopy biopsy and culture, carbon isotope urea is next test, breath test and ELISA serology.
- Treatment includes pharmacological acid reduction (90%): H_2 blockers, antacids proton-pump inhibitors like omeprazole. Avoid NSAIDs, high acid producing foods, nicotine and caffeine. One week course of PPI and amoxycillin + metronidazole is successful to eradicate *H pylori.* Operations for resultant peptic ulcer include:
  1. Proximal gastric vagotomy–15% long metronidazole term recurrence but low complications (dumping, early satiety, loop syndromes, malabsorption.
  2. Selective pyloromyotomy.
  3. Truncal vagotomy, antrectomy, gastroduodenostomy (Billroth), gastrojejunostomy (Billroth) have 1.5% recurrence rate but increased incidence of dumping, afferent/efferent loop problems. Best operation is probably selective vagotomy with Roux-en-Y reconstruction.
  4. Perforation–omental patch and peritoneal lavage when opposed laparoscopically.
  5. Pyloric stenosis is endoscopic balloon therapy and pyloroplasty or gastrojejunostomy.
- Symptoms–epigastric pain–variable relief with food/antacids–weight loss.

- Diagnosis–UGI or EGD with biopsy–most are on lesser curve near antrum–beware of those on greater curve.
- Treatment:
  1. Antacids, H_2 blockers, cytoprotective agents (sucralfate, omeprazole) along with correcting underlying mucosal injury agents are effective. Pharmacologic management has 50–60% recurrence rate for benign gastric ulcers.
     a. Must re-endoscope or UGI series after six weeks to be sure ulcer has healed.
  2. Indication for operation, hemorrhage, obstruction, perforation, with best medical management (if ulcer nor healed within 6 weeks, the ulcer need to be excised to eliminate the possibility of cancer.
  3. Operations include

Closure of perforation if perforated ulcer by distal gastrectomy
  a. Excision of ulcer–antrectomy if ulcer is distal (the ulcer must be excised).
  b. Vagotomy added if patient secretes significant acid.

- Zollinger Ellison syndrome presents with epigastric pain, resistant ulceration, diarrhea, weight loss (40% oesophagitis). Acute gastritis is characterized by edema–infiltrate leading to ischaemia and sloughing to produce acute ulcer. Menterier's disease is hypertonic gastropathy with hypochlorhydria, hypoproteinaemia, epigastric pain, diarrhoea and treatment is antisecretory drugs and partial and total gastrectomy.

POSTGASTRECTOMY SYNDROMES

Early Dumping

1. Uncontrolled dumping of hypertonic fluid into small bowel–results in acute hypovolemia and release of vasoactive hormones (serotonin, histamine, glucagon, VIP).
2. Manifested by weakness, tachycardia, diaphoresis, palpitations and occasionally diarrhea.
3. Treat by avoiding liquids with meals, avoid alcohol, ingest some fat with each meal and propanolol.

Late Dumping

1. Similar symptoms to early dumping but occurs 3–5 hours after meals
2. Due to changes in insulin and glucose levels
3. Treated by eating a small snack two hours after meals.

After Loop Syndrome

1. Occurs after Billroth II reconstruction and is associated with a kink in the afferent limb
2. Pancreatic and bile juice causes crampy pain and finally vomiting without food particles
3. Treat with conversion of Billroth II to Roux-en-Y anastomosis.

Blind Loop Syndrome

1. Bacterial overgrowth in a loop or limb of bowel which does not have chyme flowing through it
2. Interfaces with folate and vitamin B_{12} metabolism leading to anaemia
3. Treat with antibiotics.

Alkaline Reflux Gastritis

1. Weakness, weight loss, nausea, abdominal pain and anaemia due to reflux of alkaline biliary/pancreatic fluid into stomach
2. Treatment–divert biliary fluid from stomach.

Nutritional Deficiencies

1. Especially vitamin B_{12} folate iron
2. Many patients have diarrhea and weight loss.

Upper Gastrointestinal Bleeding

1. *Haematemesis is vomiting of blood:* It may be bright or look like coffee grounds. Melaena mean black motions, often like tar (signifying altered blood, which has a characteristic smell). Both indicate upper GI bleeding.
2. Causes
   a. Common
      i. Duodenal/gastric ulcer
      ii. Gastritis/gastric erosions
      iii. Mallory-Weiss tear
      iv. Duodenitis
      v. Oesophageal varices
      vi. Oesophagitis
      vii. Malignancy
      viii. Drugs (NSAIDs steroids, thrombolytics and anticoagulants).
   b. Uncommon
      i. Bleeding disorders
      ii. Portal hypertensive gastropathy
      iii. Haemobilia (bleeding in billiary tree)
      iv. Dieulafoy lesion (rupture of an usually big arteriole, e.g. in fundus)
      v. Aortoenteric fistula and angioplasty
      vi. Meckel's diverticulum
      vii. Peutz-Jeghers syndrome
      viii. OslerWeber-Rendu syndrome.
3. *Assessment:* Brief history and examination to assess severity.
4. *History:* Ask about pervious GI bleed; dyspepsia of known DU/GU, known liver disease or oesophageal varices, dysphagia, vomiting and weight loss. Check drugs (NSAIDs steroids) anticoagulants and alcohol consumption is there serious

concomitant disease, e.g. cardiovascular disease, respiratory disease. Hepatic or renal impairment, or malignancy.

5. *Examination:* Look for sign of chronic liver disease and do the check for melana. Is the patient shocked?
   (a) Peripherally shut down (cool and clammy)
   (b) Tachycardia (pulse >100 MIN, and JVP not raised)
   (c) Hypotensive (systolic BP <100 mm Hg)
   (d) Postural drop in BP
   (e) Poor urine output, e.g. <30 ml/hr
6. *Acute management:* In summary:
   (a) Protect airway and give high-flow oxygen
   (b) Insert 2 large-bore IV cannulae and take blood for FBC, clotting cross-match 4–6 units (1 unit per gm/dl <14 g/dl).
   (c) Give IV colloid (e.g. haemocoel 500–1000 ml) while waiting for blood to be cross-matched. In a dire emergency, give group O Rh –ve blood.
   (d) Insert a CVP line to monitor CVP and guide fluid replacement
   (e) Transfuse until hemodynamically stable
   (f) Correct clotting abnormalities (vitamin K, FFP platelets)
   (g) Monitor pulse, BP and CVP at least hourly until stable
   (h) Insert a urinary catheter and monitor hourly urine output
   (i) Organise a CXR, ECG and check arterial blood gases in high-risk patient
   (j) Arrange an urgent endoscopy
   (k) Notify surgeons of all sever bleeds on admission
7. Further management
   (a) Re-examine after 4 hours and give FFP if >4 units transfused
   (b) Monitor pulse, BP, CVP and urine output hourly; frequency to the haemodynamically stable
   (c) Check LFT and clotting daily
   (d) Transfuse to keep Hb >10g/dl; always keep 2 units of blood in reverse
   (e) Keep nil by mouth for 24 hrs. Allow clear fluids after 24 hrs and light diet after 28 hrs, if no evidence of rebleeding.

Upper Gastrointestinal Bleeding

1. Endoscopy should be arranged after resuscitation and adrenaline, sclerotherapy and banding can be done, varicel hemorrhage results in developing of dilated collateral veins at sites of portosystemic anastmosis found in lower esophagus, umbilicus and rectum. Management includes sclerotherapy and surgical decomposition by shunts (TIPS).

GASTRIC CANCER

Adenocarcinoma most common–rare lymphoma, leiomyosarcoma.

Associated factors same as with gastric ulcers–also achlorhydria, pernicious anemia, Barrett's esophagus and lye ingestion.

Declining incidence M : F : 2:1. High in Japan, Eastern Europe. Diet rich in nitrosamines such as meat and fish. Low socioecononic status, blood group A, pernicious anaemia, atrophic gastritis, hypogammaglobunaemia, *H. pylori* infection, postgastrectomy. Mostly adenocarcinoma classified as macroscopic appearance (Borrman's classification).

1. Fungating
2. Excavated
3. Ulcerative and raised
4. Linitis plastica

Lauren classification relies on histological classification. Early gastric cancer is limited to mucosa or submucosa. 5-year survival 95% and spread to pancreas, retroperitoneum and lymphatic. Symptoms of early gastric cancer are weight loss (20%–60%), abdominal pain (20%–90%), nausea (20%), dysphagia (25%). Diagnostic tools are double control barium meal, fibroptic endoscopy (87%), CT scan and laproscopy. The only potentially curative either subtotal gastrectomy. Treatment is surgery and adequate proximal 4 to 6 cm proximal and distal should be resected with en block D_2 resection, lymphadenectomy. In early gastric cancer adjuvant radiotherapy and chemotherapy are not recommended.

Gastric volvulus is organic-axial or along longitudinal curative axis and mesentero-axial rotation along transverse axis. Acute gastric dilatation may follow gastric or abdominal surgery, trauma causing tachycardia, hiccups and bleeding.

Foreign bodies may be swallowed by children under 3-years. Lateral X-rays and endoscopy will establish diagnosis. Oesophageal foreign bodies especially sharp have to be recovered and stomach it can left and serial X-ray performed to ensure passage. Surgery is only indicated in perforation of obstruction. Trichobezoar–composed of hair found in young women. Phytobezoar composed of vegetable material.

Gastric Carcinoid Tumors

Type 1 : Atrophic gastritis
Type 2 : MEN syndrome
Type 3 : Sporadic, malignant and metastasize to liver

Treatment <2 cm endoscopic excision >2 cm margin resection having proximal and distal 2 cm margin.

TUMOURS

Primary gastric lymphoma represents gastric malignancies and commonest site of extranodal non-Hodgkin's lymphoma 90% B cell origin.

Low grade Maltoma (mucosa associated lymphoid tumour).

High grade Maltoma: Clinical features include dyspepsia, anorexia, weight loss, anaemia, bleeding, investigations OGD and biopsy, endoluminal ultrasound and CT scan. Treatment is total or near total gastrectomy.

Late Gastric Causes

TNM staging of AJCC and UICC

T_0 No evidence

T_{IS} CA *in situ*–no invasion of lamina propria
T_1 Invasion of lamina
T_2 Invasion of muscularis propria
T_3 Invasion of serosa
T_4 Invasion of surrounding tissue
N_0 No nodal disease
N_1 1–6 nodal involved
N_2 7–15 nodes involved
N_3 15 nodes involved
M_1 Metastasis present

Stage-I	:	$T_1/T_2N_0/N_1M_0$	Early
Stage-II	:	T_1N_2, T_2N_1, $T_3N_0M_0$	Locally advanced
Stage-III	:	$T_2/T_3N_0/N_1T_3N_2M_0$	Locally advanced
Stage-IV	:	T_4/N_1M_1 any M_1	Metastasis

Diagnosis is upper GI endoscopy, endoscopic ultrasound, CT scan, MRI, laparoscopy tumor markers and peritoneal fluid cytology.

Treatment

Surgery is the only modality and minimal margin to 5 cm

Distal gastric cancer	Distal radical/total
Body gastric cancer	Total radical
Proximal gastric cancer	Extended total gastrectomy including distal esophagus

Lymphadenectomy can be

D_1 gastrectomy	Perigastric nodes along lesser or greater curvature
D_2 gastrectomy	1–6 nodes, celiac, splenic and artery
D_3 gastrectomy	Along hepatoduodenal ligament, retropancreatic and root of mesentry
D_4 gastrectomy	Lymph nodes 15–16–para-aortic and paraceliac

Paraceliac Nodes

Advanced gastric cancer there is invasion of muscularis and lymph node metasis. Treatment is Billroth II, Total gastrectomy and esophagojejunostomy proximal and distal should be clear to tumor 4–6 cm.

R_1 Excision of perigastric lymph nodes and removal of macroscopic disease.

R_2 Excision of perigastric, splenic and hepatic.

Chemotherapy used as neoadjuvant in local advanced. Wilks has used (EAP) (Etoposide + Adriamycin + **DDP**), some use 5FU + Adriamycin. Radiotherapy can be given preoperative and postoperative and as stomach is radiosensitive 4500 cGy.

QUESTIONS AND ANSWERS

1. **What are the important differential diagnoses of gastric ulcer?**
   Ans: Differential diagnosis include peptic ulcer, reflux esophagitis, gastritis symptoms gallstone disease, and ischemic heart disease.
2. **How long can portal vein and hepatic arterial flow to the liver be interrupted? What are the Pringle maneuver?**
   Ans: In the normothermic liver, blood flow can be interrupted for 15 minutes without hepatocellular damage. If prolonged control of hepatic blood flow is necessary, the occlusion can be briefly released, then reapplied every 10–15 minutes. The Pringle maneuver consists of occlusion of the portal triad (portal vein, hepatic artery and common bile duct) by placement of a vascular clamp across the hepatoduodenal ligament.
3. **What is a Sengstaken-Blakemore tube?**
   Ans: The Sengstaken-Blakemore tube consists of two balloons: One is inflated in the stomach the other in the esophagus.
4. **What is child's classification?**
   Ans: Child classification:

	A	*B*	*C*
Serum bilirubin (mg/dl)	Below 2.0	2.0–3.0	Over 3.0
Serum albumin (mg/dl)	Over 3.5	3.0–3.5	Under 3.0
Ascitis	None	Easily controlled	Poorly controlled
Neurologic disorder	None	Minimal	Advanced
Nutrition	Excellent	Good	Poor

5. **Which operations are used for emergency treatment of variceal hemorrhage?**
   Ans: The goal of emergency operation for varices hemorrhage is control of bleeding. Less concern is placed on postoperative sequelae (encephalopathy) when exsanguinations is the alternatives. A form of central (nonselective) portosystemic shunt is usually employed in the emergency setting. The most expeditious shunt is performed by placed a graft between the proximal superior mesenteric vein nd the vena cava (mesocaval shunt). Other emergent operation including direct esophageal varix ligation, splenectomy, or esophageal transaction are often only temporarily effective in controlling bleeding.
6. **What space lies behind the stomach?**
   Ans: The lesser sac, the pancreas lies behind the stomach.
7. **What is the opening into the lesser?**
   Ans: Foremen of Winslow.
8. **Define the products of the following stomach cells**
   a. Gastric parietal cells
   b. Chief cells
   c. G cells
   d. Where are G cells located?
   e. Mucosa neck cells
   a. HCl and intrinsic factor
   b. Pepsinogen
   c. Antrum
   d. Bicarbonate mucus

9. **What is intrinsic factor?**
Ans: A protein secreted by th parietal cells that combines with vitamin B_{12} and allows for absorption in the terminal ileum.

10. **What is gastroesophageal reflux disease (GERD)?**
Ans: Excessive reflux of gastric contents into the esophagus (everyone refluxes to a small degree); "heartburn".

11. **What are the causes of gastroesophageal reflux disease (GERD)?**
Ans: Decreased lower esophagus sphincter (LES) form (>50% of Disease). Decreased esophageal motility to clear refluxed fluid. Gastric outlet obstruction Hiatal hernia.

12. **What are the signs/symptoms of gastroesophageal reflux disease (GERD)?**
Ans: Heartburn, regurgitation, respiratory problems/pneumonia from aspiration of reflux gastric contents; substernal pain.

13. **What tests are included in the working?**
Ans: EGD, UGI contrast study: Twenty-four hour acid analysis (pH probe in esophagus), manometry.

14. **What is the medical treatment?**
Ans: Small meals: Omeprazole or other PPIs (proton-pump inhibitors). Elevation of head at night and no meals prior to sleeping.

15. **What are indications for surgery?**
Ans: Intractability (failure of medical treatment). Respiratory problems as a result of reflux and aspiration of gastric contents (e.g., pneumonia). Severe esophageal injury (e.g., ulcers, hemorrhage, stricture, ± Barrett's esophagus). Young age at onset.

16. **What is Barrett's esophagus?**
Ans: Columnar metaplasia from the normal squamous epithelium as a result of chronic irritation from reflux.

17. **What type of cancer develops in Barrett's esophagus?**
Ans: Adenocarcinoma.

18. **Define the following surgical options for severe gastroesophageal reflux disease (GERD)**
    (a) LAP Nissen
    (b) How does the Nissen wrap work?
    (c) What are the postoperative complications?
        a. 360° fundoplication: 2 cm long and loose (laparoscopically)
        b. Controversial but thought to work by:
        Increasing LES muscular tone
        Elongating LES
        Restoring angle of HIS
        Decreasing distal esophageal diameter may have competent wrap intrathoracic.

19. **What is the Blumer's shelf?**
Ans: A solid peritoneal deposit anterior to the rectum, forming a "shelf," palpated on rectal examination.

20. **What is the Virchow's node?**
Ans: Metastatic gastric cancer to the nodes in the left supraclavicular fossa.

21. **What is Sister Mary Joseph's sign?**
Ans: Periumbilical lymph node gastric cancer metastases presents as periumbilical mass.

22. What is a Krukenberg's tumour?
Ans: Gastric cancer (or other adenocarcinoma) that has metastasized to the ovary.

23. What is "Irish's" node?
Ans: Left axillary adenopathy from gastric cancer metastasis.

24. What is the morphology of gastric cancer?
Ans: Ulcerative (25%), polyploid (25%), superficial spreading (10%), linitis plastica(10%).

25. Which morphologic type is named after a leather bottle?
Ans: Linitis plastia–the entire stomach is involved and looks thickened.

26. What is the treatment?
Ans: Surgical resection with wide (>5 cm checked by frozen section) margins and lymph node dissection.

27. What operation is performed the tumour in the : (a) Antrum?, (b) Midbody?, (c) Proximal?
Ans: (a) Distal subtotal gastrectomy, (b) Total gastrectomy, (c) Total gastrectomy.

28. What is the differences between a subtotal gastrectomy and a hemigastrectomy?
Ans: Hemigastrectomy = 50% of stomach removed. Subtotal gastrectomy = 75% of stomach removed.

29. What type of anastomosis?
Ans: Billroth III or Roux-en-Y (never use a Billroth I).

30. When should splenectomy be performed?
Ans: When the tumor directly invades the spleen/splenic hilum or with splenic hilar adrenopathy.

31. Define extended lymph node dissection
Ans: Extensive lynph node dissection, usually one group past the lymph node group with positive metastases.

32. What is the 5-year survival rate for gastric cancer?
Ans: 10% of patients are alive 5-year diagnosis in the United States (in Japan 50% are alive at 5-year).

Flow Chart: Upper GI bleeding

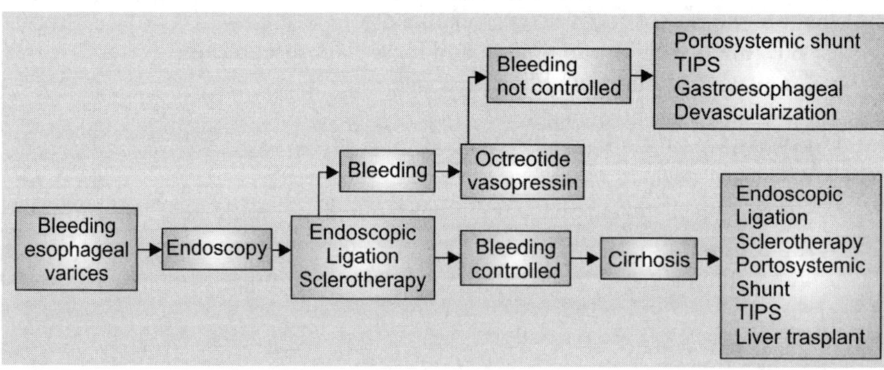

Flow Chart: Gastric ulcer

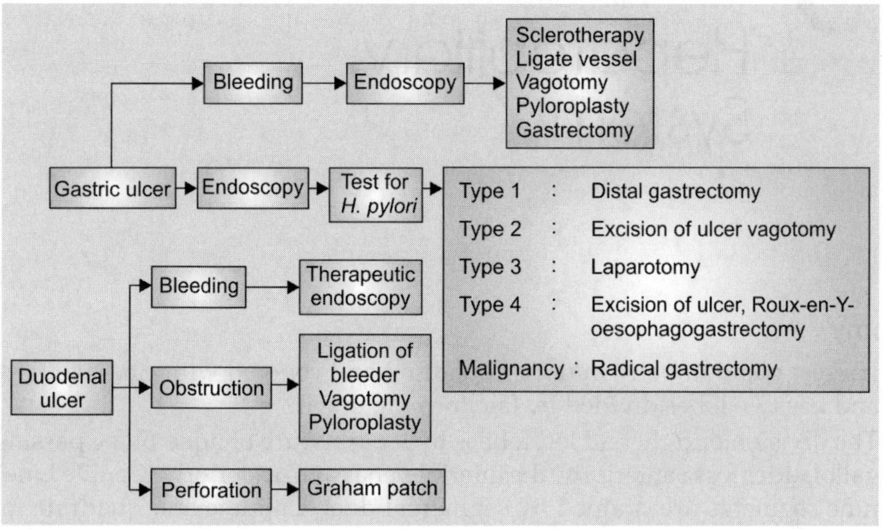

13 Hepatobiliary System

LIVER

Anatomy

- Largest gland of body in upper quadrant and covered with ribs, 1400–1800 gm and has two lobes divided by falciform ligament.
- The division of right and left lobe is by lobar fissure oblique plane passing from gallbladder fossa anteriorly, the inferior vena cava posteriorly (Cantile Line). Each nine segments are drained by segmental duct. Caudate and quadrate lobe are centrally placed.
- Portal vein (formed from the confluence of the splenic and superior mesenteric veins) enters the liver at the hilum and disperses into the portal triads (along with the hepatic artery branches and bile duct branches). Portal vein supplied 75% of hepatic blood flow but 50% of O_2 delivery.
- Hepatic artery (branch of celiac axis) supplies only 25% of blood flow but 50% of O_2 delivery via the portal triads.
- Bile duct in portal triads collect the secretions of the hepatocytes and deliver it to the right and left hepatic ducts, the proper hepatic duct and then the common bile duct.
- Blood from the portal triad vessels (portal vein and hepatic artery) the Kupffer's cells (phagocytosis of foreign bodies, bacteria, etc.) down the column of hepatocytes into the central vein. The central veins coverage and eventually lead to the right, middle and left hepatic veins which drain into the inferior vena cava.

Physiology

- Perform hemopoietic function in fetus and neonate.
- Complex hepatocellular functions severe to metabolize numerous drugs and chemicals in the body as well as serving an immunosuppressive function.

GALLBLADDER

Anatomy

- Pear shaped reservoir of bile, on inferior surface or right lobe of liver, 3–4 inches long, 30–50 cc and has fundus, corpus, infundibulum and neck. Its wall is made up of smooth muscle.
- Common bile duct (empties through ampulla of Vater)–cystic duct (lined with valves of Heister)–common hepatic duct (3" long, 6 mm diameter)–right and left hepatic ducts (1" long).

- Common hepatic artery (from celiac axis)–gastroduodenal artery and proper and right hepatic artery–cystic artery.
- Ductal and arterial anatomy is extremely variable.

Physiology

- Severe as a storage and concentrating organ of liver-produced bile (500–1200 ml/day).
- Bile in gallbladder is a balance of the concentration of bile salts, (75%) phospholipids, (lecithin) (20%) and cholesterol (5%)–abnormalities in this balance causes development of stones. Gallbladder can concentrates bile 10 times.
- Contraction stimulated by cholecystokinin (CCK) released from duodenum in response to fats and acidity. (CCK = pancreozymin).
- Ultrasound is used to assess stones and CBD diameter.

Investigations for hepatobiliary system include liver function tests, serum total protein, glucose, prothrombin time, ultrasound. IV cholangiogram, oral cholecystogram, CT scan, MRI scan, ERCP and MRCP and nuclear tests.

Obstructive jaundice is when conjugated bilirubin cannot get into gut and appears in blood and excreted in urine. Haem–unconjugated bilirubin–conjugated in liver blockage extrahepatic ducts–no stercobilinogen–pale faeces and conjugated bilirubin in blood–jaundice conjugated–bilirubin in urine.

Onset	*Type of jaundice*	*Alkaline phosphatase*	*Serum transaminase*	*Bilirubin*	*Serum albumin*
Acute obstructive		+++	+	+	Normal
	Hepatocellular	+	+++	++	Normal
Chronic	Obstructive	+++	+	+	Low
	Hepatocellular	+	+++	++	Very low

Congenital Problems

Biliary Atresia

- Varying degrees of atresia of the extrahepatic and intrahepatic ducts with prognosis inversely proportional to the degree of atresia.
- Previously treated with biliary-enteric anastomoses; now treated with liver transplants when organs available.
- Agenesis and duplication of gallbladder and ductal system have also been reported.

Calculus Associated Illnesses

Composition

1. Gall stones–bile contains cholesterol bile pigments and phospholipids. If concentration of these cholesterol vary different kind of stones may be formed. Cholesterol and lipids bile are not water soluble but have to be kept soluble to

prevent them from deposition as stone. Bile salts and lecithin are amphoteric and aggregate to form A core that carries cholesterol.

2. May be pure "pigment stones" (25%), especially associated with hemolytic disorders, i.e. sickle cell anemia, spherocytosis, etc.) may be pure cholesterol stones (most responsive of dissolution therapy), but most commonly are "mixed stones"–pigment, cholesterol, calcium and 10% gallstones are radiopaque.

Asymptomatic Stones

1. Incidence of developing symptoms is approximately 20% over lifetime; once symptoms develop they usually recur.
2. High-risk patients with asymptomatic stones (diabetes mellitus, immunosuppressed, etc.) should have gallbladder out before symptoms appear.

Acute Cholecystitis

1. Inflammatory condition of gallbladder associated with stones >90%.
2. Results from obstruction of cystic duct by stone, bacterial overgrowth with altered mucous membrane, permeability, increased secretion versus absorption, swelling of gallbladder and edema of wall, leading to congestion of lymphatic, venous and then arterial flow.
   a. Biliary colic represents repeated symptomatic episodes which spontaneously resolve (presumably because of migration of obstructing stone).
   b. Murphy sign–lay 2 fingers over right upper abdomen and ask patient to breath in. It cause pain and of inspiration as inflamed GB impinges on your fingers.
2. Clinical manifestations
   a. Present in overweight, middle aged, females, fat, fertile and female of fifty.
   b. Right upper quadrant crampy pain 30 minutes after meals heavy with greasy, fatty and spicy food.
   c. Nausea, vomiting and occasionally fever.
   d. Ultrasound very accurate at diagnosis shows thickened GB pericholecystic fluid and stones.
   e. There may be increased WBC, increased alkaline phosphatase, increased bilirubin and hepatocellular enzymes.
   f. Management includes NG suction, IV fluids resuscitation, antibiotics (cephalosporins are highly concentrated in bile–usual organisms include *E coli, Klebsiella, Enterobacter, Salmonella*) and analgesics.
   g. Operative cholecystectomy (open or laparoscopic).

Chronic cholecystitis–Stones Causes Inflammation and Colic

1. Patients have repeated, short, often self-limited bouts of biliary colic.
2. Cavosier's law: In obstruction of common bile duct due to stone distention of gallbladder seldom occurs.

3. Treatment
   a. Operative removal of gallbladder–(open or laparoscopic) laparoscopic cholecystectomy is treatment of choice.
   b. Dissolution therapy–use of chenodeoxycholic acid to dissolve the 30–40% of stones which are pure cholesterol–require months to work-high incidence of stone reformation with cessation of therapy–numerous complications of treatment especially nausea and diarrhea.
   c. Lithotripsy–use of directed ultrasound to break the stones–followed by dissolutions therapy.

Choledocholithiasis

1. 15% of patients with gallstones will have stones in the common bile duct.
2. Right upper quadrant pain with jaundice and fever (Charcot's triad) is associated with acute descending cholangitis.
3. Diagnostic work-up of jaundice associated with probable choledocholithiasis includes:
   a. Ultrasound
   b. Liver function test–magnetic resonance cholangiopancreatography.
   c. Endoscopic retrograde cholangiopancreatography (ERCP).
4. Treatment is antibiotic therapy and drainage of the biliary tree, either by percutaneous placement of a catheter or papillectomy of the common bile duct.
5. The patients with a symptomatic common bile duct stone, require operative removal.
   a. The absolute indications for exploring a common bile duct include a palpable common duct stone or common duct stones visualized on intraoperative cholangiogram.
   b. Relative indications include bile duct dilatation, jaundice, history of gallstone pancreatitis, multiple small stone and a single, multifaceted gallstone.
6. After exploration of the common bile duct, postoperative drainage through a T-tube is important because of a small chance of residual stones after exploration.
7. The operative mortality to cholecystectomy and common bile duct exploration may be as much as 8–10 percent.
8. Laparoscopic cholecystectomy with primary closure and stone removal its becoming popular.
9. Ideal treatment is ERCP for removal of CBD stone followed by lap cholecystectomy.

Gallstone Associated Pancreatitis

1. Occurs when a stone passes through ampulla of Vater, causing edema of orifice or pancreatic duct when pancreas is actively secreting. Usually do not find an impact stone in the duct but can find stone in the stool.
2. Clinical manifestations similar to acute cholecystitis but with elevated serum amylase and epigastric, pain to radiating to back. Requires cholecystectomy and ERCP or surgical removal of common bile duct stones.
3. After amylase has decreased and patients clinical symptoms have resolved.

Gallstone Ileus

1. Small bowel obstruction caused by a large gallstone which has eroded into duodenum (or occasionally jejunum) and becomes lodged in the small bowel (usually distal ileum).
2. Required removal of the stone and gallbladder as well as repair of the biliary-enteric fistula.

Cancer

Common Bile Duct

1. Adenocarcinoma may occur in any area of the bile duct but most commonly involves the extrahepatic ducts. Etiology unknown, but associated with stones in 60%.
   a. Other diseases associated with increased incidence of bile duct cancer include choledochal cysts, Charcot's disease and ulcerative colitis.
2. Patients are between 50 and 70 years and present with weight loss and painless obstructive jaundice and abnormal mass.
3. Ultrasound of liver reveals dilated ducts serum bilirubin is remarkably raised >10 mg/dl. CT scan can also help identify intrahepatic lesions and metastasis to nearby lymph nodes. Occasionally ERCP will be able to see tumor and biopsy it. MRCP is done as noninvasive investigation bile duct stones for common. Hilar cholangiocarcinoma, Klatskin tumor is present in 8% cases. Proximal 15% and middle third 27% tumors are amneble to Roux-en-Y hepaticojejunostomy. In distal third 10% and periampullary 37% resection is greater than 50%.
4. Treatment is total excision, if possible, (often requiring a Whipple procedure). Bypass operation or Stents if cure seems unlikely. Total removal carries a 30–40% 5-year survival. Chemotherapy and radiation are not very effective at this time.

Adenocarcinoma of Gallbladder

Carcinoma gallbladder fifth most common malignancy occurring above 65 years.

1. Not sensitive to radiation or chemotherapy, so wide local excision is the treatment of choice with good, long-term prognosis if tumor completely removed. Usually, however, has metastasized before detection, leading to an overall 5-year survival of <5%.
2. Calcification of gallbladder wall (porcelain gallbladder) has a 60% association with gallbladder cancer. Symptoms are weight loss, anorexia, jaundice, treatment is radical cholecystectomy with anterior wedge resection of segment IV liver and lymph node dissection.

Congenital Abnormalities

- Most surgical important congenital problems involve atresia of biliary tract.
- Numerous congenital or genetic abnormalities of hepatic function may lead to the need for hepatic transplant, Gaucher's disease, Wilson's disease.

Inflammatory Problems

Bacterial

1. Pyogenic hepatic abscesses gain access to the liver via the biliary or portal venous system; most commonly involve enteric bacilli (*E. coli*, *Klebsiella*, *Serratia*, *Salmonella*, etc.) and originate with cholangitis, appendicitis, diverticulitis or occasionally salpingitis.
2. Patient present with fever, right upper quadrant pain, +/- jaundice, CT scan and U/S are useful in localizing abscesses as well.
3. The source of infection, intrahepatic abscesses should be drained if possible either operatively or now more commonly through percutaneously placed catheters, and treated with appropriate antibiotics and mortality 10–40%.

Amoebic Abscesses

1. Eosinophilia may accompany increased WBC, fever, etc.
2. Usually can be treated with antibiotics with good results (Metronidazole).
3. "Anchovy paste"–like material in cavity.
4. Occurs without amoebic dysentery in 50% of cases.

Echinococcus Cyst

1. Caused by echinococcus granulosus–usually, accompanies concomitant pulmonary disease–usually solitary and often calcified cyst in right lobe of liver. Clinical features are palpable mass, pain and fever intermittent with chills.
2. Eosinophilia present 30%, indirect agglutination test is 85% and positive casoni test in 90%.
3. Attempt to sterilize cyst by injection of hypertonic saline prior to excision or external drainage.
4. Important to avoid intra-abdominal spread. Treatment is surgical excision.

Sclerosing Cholangitis

1. Usually presents in 3rd–4th decade as sepsis problems related to multiple intrahepatic abscesses.
2. ERCP reveals multiple sclerotic bile ducts (intra-and extrahepatic) with numerous abscess cavities in both lobes of the liver.
3. Etiology is thought to be autoimmune (associated with ulcerative colitis).
4. Treatment involves drainage of abscesses, antibiotics and transplantation when possible. Laparoscopic and open drainage is mainstay of treatment of liver abscesses. Portal hypertension occurs when portal venous pressure exceeds hepatic venous pressure by 8 mm Hg. Normal portal venous pressure 10 mm Hg.

Portal Hypertension

Etiology

Portal hypertension occurs when portal venous pressure exceeds hepatic venous pressure by 8 mm Hg portal veins have no valves. Increases in pressures causes varices at sites of portosystemic anastomosis.

1. Prehepatic–portal vein occlusion (common in infants and children) or splenic vein occlusion (usually secondary to pancreatitis or trauma), associated with normal liver function.
2. Intrahepatic–alcohol induced cirrhosis most common in United States, also post-hepatitis (post-necrotic) cirrhosis and intrahepatic infections or metabolic problems which lead to obstruction of portal venous flow directly or indirectly via scarring (cirrhosis).
3. Posthepatic–hepatic vein occlusion (Budd-Chiari syndrome) due to hypercoagulable state or tumor growth and obstruction of hepatic veins (hypernephroma) associated with severe ascites.
4. Collateral venous decompression of elevated portal pressures occurs through (a) Coronary vein/Esophageal varices, (b) Periumblical veins (Caput Medusa), (c) Superior hemorrhoidal, (d) Veins of Retzius, (e) Veins of Sappey.

Clinical Manifestations and Management

1. Upper GI bleeding due to enlarged esophageal or gastric varices is the most common manifestation.
   a. 75% of patients will re-bleed in one year and 60% will die in the one year.
   b. Initial treatment includes IV fluid and coagulation defect correction, gastric lavage, IV Pitressin, esophagogastric balloon tamponade (Sengstaken-Blackemore tube).
   c. Early endoscopy and sclerotherapy (effective) in stopping initial hemorrhage in 85–90%.
   d. Long-term management includes sclerotherapy at regular intervals (problems with ulceration, stricture and development of gastric varices), portosystemic shunts (portocaval or mesocaval H-grafts) (5–10% perioperative mortality, 5% re-bleed rate, 20–30% encephalopathy rate), selective shunting (distal splenorenal shunt 5% perioperative mortality, 10% re-bleed rate, 5 encephalopathy rate) TIPS procedures (transjugular intrahepatic portosystemic shunt), esophageal transaction and liver esophageal transections and transplantation.
   e. Perioperative prognosis predicted on basis of hepatic function. Child's classification

	A	B	C
Bilirubin	<2.0	2.0–3.0	>3.0
Albumin	>3.5	3.0–3.5	<3.0
Ascites	None	Easily controlled	Not controlled
Encephalopathy	None	Minimum	Advanced
Nutrition	Excellent	Good	Poor
Mortality	5%	10%	40%

a. Ascites usually a prominent feature of patients with hepatic vein occlusion (Budd-Chiari) and often of patients with intrahepatic cirrhosis, but ascites does not generally form in patients with portal vein occlusion.
b. Most ascites can be controlled with bed rest, sodium restriction and gentle diuresis (Spironolactone). Peritoneal–venous shunts can be helpful but can thrombose on induce a consumptive coagulopathy or lead to pulmonary edema. Portosystemic shunt (portocaval or mesocaval) are occasionally done to relieve severe ascites.

Neoplasia

Benign

1. Hepatic adenomas (associated with birth control pills), focal nodular hyperplasia and hemangiomas are the most common. Ultrasonography will show CT scan show hypodense lesions.
2. These usually do not require any treatment unless they grow to very large size, rupture, or cause pain, in which cases they are removed. Wedge resection may suffise but hepatic lobectomy may be required in selected cases.

Malignant

1. Most common malignancy in liver is metastatic disease from other primary sites; especially colon.
2. Resection of isolated metastatic lesions (especially from colon carcinoma) can increase survival.
3. Primary hepatomas are relatively unusual but more common in oriental populations.
   a. Three main types are hepatoma, cholangiocarcinoma or mixed type:
      i. Related to cirrhosis, hepatitis B, C, alpha-1 antitrypsin deficiency and hemochromatosis.
   b. Diagnosis can be made when a tender hepatic mass is identified on exam, localized by CT and often evaluated for possible resection with arteriogram.
   c. Treatment involves resection when possible. These tumors are fairly resistant to chemotherapy and radiation therapy.
   d. Hepatocellular cancers are one of the commonest cancers. Risk factor include Hepatitis-B carrier (90%), aflatoxin B. Clinical features are pain, jaundice, mass in abdomen. Diagnosis is liver function tests, alpha fetoprotein ultrasound and CT scans, alpha fetoprotein, treatment–HCC is not radio or chemoresistant. Neoadjuvant chemotherapy, transarterial chemoimbolization, cryotherapy have been tried. Surgical resection is mainstay of treatment. Right and left hemihepatectomy with preservation of caudate lobe, extended right hemihepatectomy (leaving segment I, II, III) or segmentectomies operative morbidity is 5% with 25–50% 5-year survival. Radiofrequency ablation is treatment in smaller tumours.

QUESTIONS AND ANSWERS

1. **What oral agents are used for gallstone dissolution and how do they work?**
Ans: Chenodeoxycholic acid and ursodeoxycholic acid have been demonstrated to be equally efficacious in dissolving cholesterol gallstones when taken chronically (over 6 months). Chenodeoxycholate, a primary bile salt, lowers the bile cholesterol saturation and ursodeoxycholate affects cholesterol solubilization. Recurrence of stones with discontinuation of the drug is a significant problem.
2. **How does acalculous cholecystitis differ from that of calculous cholecystitis?**
Ans: Instead of gallstones, a functional obstruction causes blockage of the outlet of the gallbladder. Associated with disease states such as burns, trauma, sepsis, major operations, and chronic total parenteral nutrition, acalculous cholecystitis is through to occur as a result of decreased gallbladder contractions (causing stasis of bile), ischemia of the gallbladder wall (causing gangrene and necrosis), and sepsis (endotoxin-mediated cholecystitis). Perhaps the most significant distinction is that acalculous cholecystitis has a high incidence of gangrene and perforation, and because these usually occur in patients who are already severely ill, the association morbidity and mortality are high.
3. **What is Hartmann's pouch?**
Ans: Gallbladder infundibulum.
4. **What are boundaries of triangle of Calot?**
Ans:
Cystic duct
Common hepatic duct
Cystic artery
5. **What is in bile?**
Ans: Cholesterol, lecithin, bile acids and bilirubin
6. **Where are most of bile acids absorbed?**
Ans: Terminal ileum.
7. **What are origins of obstructive jaundice?**
Ans: Jaundice, dark urine, clay colored stools, pruritis, loss of appetite and nausea.
8. **What causes itching in obstructive jaundice?**
Ans: Bile salts in dermis.
9. **Define the following studies.**
Ans: ERCP–Endoscopic retrograde cholangiopancreatography.
Radioisotope scanning for cholecystitis (100% sensitivity). There is nonopacification of gallbladder.
10. **What is Courvoisier's law?**
Ans: In an obstructive jaundice due to common bile duct stone is not associated with dilated gallbladder.
11. **What is timing of surgery in acute cholecystitis?**
Ans: In acute cholecystitis surgery is performed in first 24 hours when patients hemodynamic and electrolyte abnormalities corrected.
12. **What are contraindications for laparoscopic cholecystectomy?**
Ans: Pregnancy, bleeding and diathesis.

13. **Who performed first cholecystectomy care?**
Ans: Langenbuch performed first open cholecystectomy 1882 and Eric Muhe 1985 performed first laparoscopic cholecystectomy.
14. **What is Kocher manoeuvre?**
Ans: Kocher manoeuvre is done by incising lateral peritoneal reflection of second portion of duodenum.
15. **What is normal secretion of bile?**
Ans: Bile is between 250 ml and 1000 ml.
16. **What is Charcot's triad?**
Ans: Fever with chills
Abdominal pain
Jaundice
17. **What is Cholelithiasis?**
Ans: The formation of gallstones.
18. **What are the "Big-4" risk factors?**
Ans: The "Four Fs": Female, Fat, Forty, Fertile (multiparity).
19. **What are other less common risk factors for gallstones?**
Ans: Oral contraceptives, bile stasis, chronic hemolysis (pigment stones), cirrhosis, infection, rapid weight loss, obesity, inflammatory bowel disease (IBD), terminal ileal resection, total parenteral nutrition (TPN), vagotomy, advanced age, hyperlipidemia and somatostatin therapy.
20. **What is the pathogenesis of cholesterol stones?**
Ans: Secretion of bile supersaturated with cholesterol (relatively decreased amounts of lecithin and bile salts); then, cholesterol precipitates out and forms solid crystals, then gallstones.
21. **What is Boas sign?**
Ans: The referred right subscapular pain of biliary colic.
22. **What is gallstone ileus?**
Ans: Small bowel obstruction from a large gallstone (>2.5 cm) that has eroded through the gallbladder and into the duodenum/small bowel.
23. **What is carcinoma of the gallbladder?**
Ans: Malignant neoplasm arising the gallbladder; very low incidence, vast majority are adenocarcinoma (90%).
24. **What are the risk factors?**
Ans: Gallstones (approximately 100% of cases, especially large gallstones), cholecystenteric fistula, porcelain gallbladder (approximately 50% will have gallbladder cancer).
25. **What is cholangiocarcinoma?**
Ans: Malignancy of the extrahepatic or intrahepatic ducts–primary bile duct cancer.
26. **What are the sign and symptoms of cholangiocarcinoma?**
Ans: The signs and symptoms of biliary obstruction: jaundice, pruritis, dark, urine and clay-colored stools.
27. **What is a Klatskin tumor?**
Ans: Tumor that involves that junction of the right and left hepatic ducts.
28. **What are the diagnostic tests of choice?**
Ans: Ultrasound, CT, ERCP/PTC with biopsy/brushings for cytology.

29. **What is the management of cholangiocarcinoma?**
Ans: Resection with Roux-en-Y hepaticojejunostomy (anastomoses bile duct to jejunum).
30. **What is the management of distal common bile duct cholangiocarcinoma?**
Ans: Calcified gallbladder seen on abdominal X-ray; results from chronic cholelithiasis/cholecystitis with calcified scar tissue in gallbladder wall; cholecystectomy required because of the strong association of gallbladder carcinoma with this condition.
31. **What is hydrops of the gallbladder?**
Ans: Complete obstruction of the cystic duct by a gallstone, with filling of the gallbladder with fluid (not bile) form the gallbladder mucosa.
32. **What is the name of the liver capsule?**
Ans: Glisson's capsule.
33. **What is the Bare area?**
Ans: The posterior section of the liver against the diaphragm that is "bare" without peritoneal covering.
34. **What is Cantle's line?**
Ans: A line drawn between the gallbladder to just left of the inferior vena cava that transects the liver into the right and left lobes.
35. **Which ligament goes from the anterior abdominal wall to the liver?**
Ans: Falciform ligament (contains the ligament teres, which is the obliterated umbilical vein).
36. **What is the coronary ligament?**
Ans: The peritoneal reflection on top of the liver that crowns (hence "coronary") the liver and attaches it to the diaphragm.
37. **What are the triangular ligaments of the liver?**
Ans: The right and left lateral extent of the coronary ligament, which form triangles.
38. **What is the venous supply of liver?**
Ans: Portal vein (formed from the splenic vein and the superior mesenteric vein).
39. **What is the hepatic venous supply?**
Ans: Via the hepatic veins, which drain into the IVC (three veins; left, middle and right).
40. **From what sources does the liver receive blood?**
Ans: Portal system –75%, hepatic artery system –25%.
41. **What is the maximum amount of the liver that can be resected while retaining adequate liver function?**
Ans: More than 80%; if given adequate recovery time, the original mass can be regenerated.
42. **Which live enzymes are made by hepatocytes?**
Ans: AST and ALT (aspartate aminotransferase and alanine aminotransferase)
43. **What is the source of alkaline phosphates?**
Ans: Ductal epithelium (thus, elevated with ductal obstruction).
44. **How can the criteria comprising the Child's classification be remembered?**
Ans: Acronym: "A BEAN":
A Ascites
B Bilirubin
E Encephalopathy
A Albumin
N Nutrition

45. Define child's classification–A, B and C.

	Bilirubin	*Albumin*	*Nutrition*	*Encephalopathy*	*Ascites*
A	<2	>3.5	Excellent	None	None
B	2–3	3–3.5	Good	Minimal	Easily controlled
C	>3	<3	Poor	Severe	Poor controlled

Think, as in a letter grading system. A is better than B and B is better than C.

46. What is the most common live cancer?
Ans: Metastatic disease outnumbers primary tumors 20 : 1. Primary site is usually the GI tract.

47. What is the most common primary malignant liver tumor?
Ans: Hepatocellular carcinoma (hepatoma).

48. What is the most common primary benign live tumor?
Ans: Hemangioma.

49. What lab tests comprise the work-up for liver metastasis?
Ans: (AST and alkaline phosphates are most useful), CEA for suspected primary colon cancer.

50. What is the right hepatic lobectomy?
Ans: Removal of the right lobe of the liver (i.e., all tissue to the right of Cantle's line is removed).

51. What is the left hepatic lobectomy?
Ans: Removal of the left lobe of the liver (i.e., all tissue to the right of Cantle's line is removed).

52. What is a right trisegmentectomy?
Ans: Removal of all the liver tissue to the right of the falciform ligament.

53. What are the three common types of primary benign liver tumors?
Ans: (a) Hemangioma, (b) Hepatocellular adenoma, (c) Focal nodular hyperplasia.

54. What are the four common types of primary malignant liver tumors?

a. Hepatocellular carcinoma (hepatoma).
b. Cholangiocarcinoma (intrahepatic).
c. Angiosarcoma (associated with vinyl chloride, arsenic, or thorotrast contrast exposure).
d. Hepatoblastoma (most common in infants and children).

55. What is a hepatoma?
Ans: Hepatocellular carcinoma.

56. What is hepatocellular carcinoma?
Ans: Most common primary malignancy of the liver.

57. What is its incidence?
Ans: Accounts for 80% of all primary malignant liver tumors.

58. What are the associated risk factors?
Ans: Hepatitis B virus, cirrhosis, aflatoxin (fungi toxin of *Aspergillus flavus*); other risk factors; alpha-1-antityrpsin deficiency, hemochromatosis, liver fluke, clonorchis, stenosis, anabolic, steroid, poly vinyl chloride and glycogen storage disease (Type-I).

59. What are the signs/symptoms of hepatocellular carcinoma?
Ans: Dull right upper quadrant pain, hepatomegaly (classic presentation; painful hepatomegaly), abdominal mass, weight loss, paraneoplastic syndromes, signs of portal hypertension, ascites, jaundice, fever, anemia splenomegaly.

60. What tests should be ordered?
Ans: Ultrasound, CT, angiography and tumor marker elevation.

61. What is the tumor marker?
Ans: Elevated alpha-fetoprotein.

62. What is the most common way to get a tissue diagnosis?
Ans: Needle biopsy with CT, ultrasound or laparoscopic guidance.

63. What is the most common site of metastasis?
Ans: Lungs

64. What is the treatment of hepatocellular carcinoma?
Ans: Urgical resection, if possible (e.g., lobectomy); liver transplant, percutaneous ethanol tumor injection, liquid nitrogen cryotherapy and intra-arterial chemotherapy are other options.

65. What is a liver abscess?
Ans: Abscess (collection of pus) in the liver parenchyma.

66. What are the types of liver abscess?
Ans: Pyogenic (bacterial), parasitic (amebic) and fungal.

67. What is the most common location of abscess in the liver?
Ans: Right lobe > left lobe.

68. What are the sources of liver abscess?
Ans: Direct spread from biliary tract infection or portal spread from GI infection (e.g., appendicitis, diverticulitis), systemic source (bacteremia), liver trauma (e.g., liver gunshot wound) and cryptogenic (unknown source).

69. What are the two most common types?
Ans: Bacterial (most common in the United States) and amoebic (most common worldwide).

70. What are the three most common bacterial organisms affecting the liver?
Ans: Gram-negatives: *E. coli*, *Klebsiella*, and *Proteus*.

71. What is the etiology?
Ans: *Entamoeba histolytica* (typically reaches liver via portal vein from intestinal amoebiasis).

72. Classic description of abscess contents.
Ans: "Anchovy paste" pus.

73. Describe drainage of blood from the superior hemorrhoidal vein.
Ans: To the IMV, the splenic vein, and then the portal vein.

74. Where does the portal vein begin?
Ans: At the confluence of the splenic vein and the SMV.

75. What level of portal pressure is normal?
   a. Umbilical vein
   b. Coronary vein to esophageal venous plexus
   c. Retroperitoneal veins (veins of Retzius)
   d. Diaphragm veins (veins of Sappey)
   e. Superior hemorrhoidal vein to middle and inferior hemorrhoidal veins and then to the iliac vein
   f. Splenic veins to the short gastric veins.

76. What level of portal pressure is normal?
Ans: About 6 mm Hg (>10 mm Hg).

77. What is the most common cause of portal hypertension in the United States?
Ans: Cirrhosis (>90% of case).

78. What is hydatid liver cysts?
Ans: Usually a right lobe cyst filled with *Echinococcus granulosus*.

79. How is the diagnosis made?
Ans: Indirect hemagglutination antibody test (serologic testing), Casoni skin test, ultrasound, CT, radiographic imaging.

80. What is the risk of surgical removal of echinococcal (hydatid) cysts?
Ans: Rupture or leakage of cyst contents into the abdomen may cause a fatal anaphylactic reaction.

81. What is the treatment of hydatid liver cysts?
Ans: Mebendazole, followed by surgical resection; large cysts can be drained and then injected with toxic irrigant.

82. What is hemobilia?
Ans: Blood draining via the common bile duct into the duodenum.

83. What are the causes?
Ans: Trauma, percutaneous transhepatic cholangiography (PTC), tumors.

84. What is the treatment hemobilia?
Ans: Embolization of the bleeding vessel.

85. What are the association clinical findings is portal hypertension (4).
a. Caput medusa (engorgement of periumbilical veins)
b. Hemorrhoids
c. Splenomegaly
d. Esophageal varices.

86. How is portal pressure measured?
Ans: Indirect hepatic vein wedge pressure.

87. What is the etiology?
Ans: Cirrhosis (90%), schistosomiasis, hepatitis, Budd-Chiari syndrome, hemochromatosis, Wilson's disease, portal vein thrombosis, tumors, splenic vein thrombosis.

88. What is Budd-Chiari syndrome?
Ans: Thrombosis of the hepatic veins.

89. What is the most feared complication of portal hypertension?
Ans: Bleeding from esophageal varices (up to 50% mortality).

90. What are esophageal varices?
Ans: Engorgement of the esophageal venous plexus secondary to increased collateral blood flow from the portal system as a result of portal hypertension.

91. What is the "rule of two-thirds" of portal hypertension?
Ans: Two-thirds of patients with cirrhosis will develop portal hypertension. Two-thirds of patients with portal hypertension will develop esophageal varices. Two-thirds of patients with esophageal varices will bleed from the varices.

92. In patients with cirrhosis and known varices who are suffering from upper GI bleeding, how often does that bleeding result from varices?
Ans: Only about 50% of the time.

93. What are the signs/symptoms?
Ans: Hematemesis, melaena, hematochezia.

94. What is the initial treatment of variceal bleeding?
Ans: As with all upper GI bleeding; large bore IVS × 2, IV fluid, Foley catheter, NG, tube and cross blood, send labs and correct coagulpathy (vitamin K, fresh frozen plasma).

95. What is the diagnostic test of choice?
Ans: EGD (upper GI endoscopy) Remember, bleeding is the result of varices only half the time; must rule out ulcers, etc.

96. If esophageal varices bleeding, what is the initial treatment?
Ans: Emergent endoscopic sclerotherapy: A sclerosing substance is injected into the esophageal varices under direct endoscopic vision.

97. What is a Sengstaken-Blackemore tube?
Ans: A tube with a gastric and esophageal balloon for tamponading an esophageal bleed.

98. What are the optics if sclerotherapy and conservative methods fail to stop the variceal bleeding or bleeding recurs?
Ans: Sclerotherapy and treat conservatively, TIPS, surgical shunt and liver transplantation.

99. What is the preferred shunt in the following cases?

A. Patient who is a candidate for liver transplant or a very poor operative candidate?
B. Nonalcoholic patient who is not a transplant candidate?
C. Patient who is an alcoholic and a good operative candidate, but not a liver transplant candidate?

A. TIPS procured
B. Warren selective shunt (distal splenorenal shunt)
C. Patient shunt: Portocaval synthetic H-graft.

100. What does the acronym TIPS stand for?
Ans: Transjugular intrahepatic portosystemic shunt.

101. What is a TIPS procedure
Ans: An angiographic radiologist places a small tube Stent intrahepatically between the hepatic vein and a branch of the portal vein via a percutaneous-jugular vein route.

102. What is Warren shunt?
Ans: Distal splenorenal shunt with ligation of the coronary vein-elective shunt procedure associated with low incidence of encephalopathy in nonalcoholic patients postoperatively because only the splenic flow is diverted to decompress the varies.

103. Define the following shunts

A. End-to-side portocaval shunt
B. Side-to-side portocaval shunt
C. Synthetic portocaval H-graft
D. Synthetic mesocaval H-graft

A. "Total shunt"–portal vein (end) to IVC (side)
B. Side of portal vein anastomosed to side of IVC–partially preserve portal flow ("partial shunt")
C. "Partial shunt"–synthetic tube graft from the portal vein to the IVC (good option for patient with alcholism; associated with lower incidence of encephalopathy and easier transplantation later)
D. Synthetic graft from the SMV to the IVC.

14

Pancreas

ANATOMY

A. Double gland both endocrine and exocrine 6–8 inches, 90 gm weight and divided into head, neck, body tail drained by pancreatic duct, 3 mm and receive tributaries.
B. Bounded on right by duodenum, left by spleen, anteriorly by stomach and transverse mesocolon and posteriorly by common bile duct, aorta, IVC, SMA/V at level of L1 and L2 vertebrae.
C. Arterial supply from gastroduodenal artery, splenic artery and gastroepiploic arteries. Venous and lymphatic drainage follow arterial routes.
D. Histologic anatomy includes ductal cells, acini cells and islets of Langerhans.
E. Vagus (parasympathetic and splanchnic (sympathetic) supply pancreas through plexus.

PHYSIOLOGY

1. Serous gland made of tubular acini lined by pyramidal cells.
2. Secretion of 1000–5000 ml/day of fluid, pH 8, chymotrypsinogen, trypsinogen, lipase, amylase, carboxypeptidase–all for digestion of proteins carbohydrates and fats after stimulates fat, protein and acid in duodenum.
3. Cholecytokinin and secretion are released from duodenal mucosa in response to amino acid fats or acid increase the enzymes in pancreatic juice, secretion, stimulates flow of HCO_3 rich water and electrolytes.

Endocrine

1. Formed by islets of Langerhans distributed a isolated masses around 2 lakh to 17 lakh and mostly in tail.
2. Inches insulin (beta cells 80%), glucagon (alpha cells 20%), gastrin (delta cells) and others.

INFLAMMATORY CONDITIONS

A. Acute inflammatory process of pancreas with pain, tenderness, vomiting and systemic inflammatory responses.
B. Acute pancreatitis
   1. Most commonly related to ETOH (ethyl alcohol) (40%)–induced ductal and parenchymal cell injury.

2. Also commonly associated with passage of gallstones past ampulla of Vater.
3. Other etiologies include trauma, hypertriglyceridemia medications, (HCTA, steroids, lasix, estrogens) Type I, IV and V hyperlipoproteinemia, familial and postoperative ischemia.
4. Causes–GET SMASHED
   a. Gallstones, ethanol (40%), trauma, steroids, mumps, autoimmune, scorpion venom, hyperlipidaemia and hyperproteinemia, ERCP drugs (azathioprine, lasix, asparagines, pentamidine, mercaptopurine and pregnancy).
   b. Pathogens–obstruction and hypersecretion and metabolic causes.
5. Manifested by epigastric abdominal pain boring through to back with fever, nausea, vomiting and elevated serum amylase and lipase levels. Sitting forward helps.
   a. Cullen's sign (periumbilical hematoma) or Grey Turner's sign (flank hematoma, local/general tenderness) suggests hemorrhagic pancreatitis.
6. Tests
   a. Serum amylase >1000 U/ml (lesser rises in cholecystitis, mesenteric infarction, GI perforation, renal failure and highest in 1st 24 hrs.
   b. Blood gases, serum lipase increase is diagnostic
   c. Abdominal films–no psoas shadow and sentinel loop of proximal jejunum
   d. CT scan and ultrasound abdomen.
7. Monitoring
   a. Hourly pulse, BP urine output, fasting blood sugar and C reaction protein
   b. ERCP–sphincterotomy indicated for gallstone pancreatitis.
8. Initial treatment includes NG suction, IV fluids–0.9% saline/haemocoel, nutrition, analgesia and possibly somatostatin to decrease exocrine function.
   a. Surgery usually reserved for complications.
9. Complications include: Early shock, renal failure and DIC
   a. Pancreatic necrosis and abscess–manifested by fever, increased WBC and persistent pain, gas on abdominal X-ray or CT scan (diffuse parenchyma). Require drainage, antibiotics and nutrition. Drainage may be laparoscopic or open, surgical drainage better than percutaneous drainage.
   b. Pseudocyst–due to leakage of a pancreatic duct and manifested by continued pain and mass. Those below 2 cm often resolve spontaneously. Larger ones or those that do not resolve spontaneously. Larger ones or those that do not resolve are allowed to "mature" for 6 weeks and then internally drainaged into the stomach or a Roux-en-Y limb of jejunum. Has a fibrous lining and epithelium.
   c. Pancreatic ascites–leakages of ductal contents into abdominal cavity; does not respond to usual treatment of ascites; needs internal drainage.
   d. Hemorrhagic pancreatitis–erosion into surrounding vessels can lead to pseudoaneurysms, massive bleeding or massive retroperitoneal bleeding and necrosis.

e. Other complications include pancreatic fistulae, pulmonary insufficiency, eventual pancreatic endocrine and exocrine dysfunction, etc.

10. Prognosis of acute pancreatitis is best estimated by Ranson's criteria (which do not include level of serum amylase).

Ranson on admission	*After 48 hours*
Age >55	Full in haematocrit–10%
WBC >16,000	Increase in bun–5 mg%
LDH >3500 IU/L	Arterial O_2 <60 mm Hg
Aspartate >250 IU/L	Base deficit >4 mmol/L
Glucose >200 mg/dl	

Management–IV fluids, plasma expanders, analgesia antibiotics, octreotide, somatostatin.

a. Ranson's criteria
b. Modified Glasgow criteria for predicting severity of pancreatitis WBC >15 × 10L, Glucose >10 mmol/L, LDH >600 IU/L, AST >200 IU/L, serum urea >16 mmol/L, serum albumin <32 gm/L, PO_2 <8 kPa. Ranson's criteria are valid for alcohol induced pancreatitis only.
c. Reactive protein–at admission: age >55; WBC >16K; glucose >200; LDH >350; SGOT >250. During 48 hours after admission: HCt >10 point decrease, BUN >5 increase; Ca^{++} <8.0; PO_2 <60 mm Hg base excess >4 mEq/L fluid sequestration >6000 ml.
d. Mortality 20% with 3–4 signs, 40% with 5–6 signs, 100% if 7 or more signs.

C. Chronic pancreatitis: Continuing irreversible pancreatitis inflammation
1. Similar etiology to cause pancreatitis but marked by endocrine/exocrine dysfunction (diabetes mellitus/steatorrhea) and calcifications in pancreas on abdominal X-rays. CT scan investigation of choice shows morphology and pancreas become hard and fibrotic distended duct.
2. Chronic pain syndrome is investigated with ERCP and treated with internal drainage of dilated obstructed duct (sphincterotomy or Puestow pancreaticojejunostomy) or pancreatic resection. Whipple operation of pancreas if body of pancreas, if body pancreas affected. Distal pancreatectomy if limited to body/tail of pancreas.

NEOPLASMS

A. Pancreatic carcinoma
1. Increasing incidence, 60–70 days in developed countries.
2. Pathology–ductal adenocarcinoma (90%), periampullary and mucinous/serous cyst adenocarcinoma.

B. Non islet cell (ductal adenocarcinoma)
1. Ductal adenocarcinoma is most common–often multicentric, associated with cigarette smoking and perhaps ETOH.

2. Occur at any location in pancreas–those in tail and body (1/3) are often far advanced prior to any symptoms. Those in the head (2/3) often lead to painless obstruction jaundice.
3. Evaluate with CT scan, PTC and ERCP.
4. Treated with excision when possible with 5% five-year survival in the 10–20% which can be resected for cure (whipple procedure) whipple–proximal pancreatoduodenectomy removes distal stomach, CBD, pancreatic head and duodenum en bloc and reconstruction with splenectomy for tumours of body and tail. Adenocarcinoma rarely resectable. Not very responsive to chemotherapy or radiation treatment.
5. Cyst adenocarcinoma may mimic pseudocyst but has an epithelial radiation lining 4000–6000 cGy and requires total excision.

C. Islet cell tumours
1. Gastrinoma, insulinoma, VIPoma and other functional tumours of APUD cell division.
2. Gastrinoma associated with Zollinger-Ellison syndrome of hyperacidity, unresponsive to further acid output stimulation, resulting in diffuse peptic ulceration in-stomach, duodenum and occasionally small bowel.
   a. Marked by increased basal acid output, no increase in acid with stimulation, increased serum gastrin levels, paradoxic decrease in gastrin with IV secretin (secretin stimulation test).
   b. Associated with MEN I syndrome (pituitary and parathyroid adenomas).
   c. Tumours from delta cells are often very small and may be multicentric but are not usually histologically malignant.
   d. If symptoms are not controlled with H_2 blockers, laparotomy indicated to try to remove tumour or do relieve symptoms. Severe or recurrent disease usually treated with total gastrectomy.
3. Insulinoma–associated with whipple triad of symptoms of hypoglycemia, with fasting low blood sugar (<50%) and relief of symptoms with glucose.
   a. Caused by a benign adenoma, occasionally localized with CT scan, MR or arteriography.
   b. On-line blood glucose determinations helpful during resection to assure removal of the tumour
   c. VIPomas–vasointestinal peptides–neuroendocrine derived tumor causing a watery diarrhea, flushing and tachycardia. Relieved by tumor excision.

TNM classification of pancreatic cancer

T_0 No evidence of pancreatic cancer
T_1 Tumor to pancreas 2 cm or less
T_2 Tumor >2 cm
T_3 Tumor extends beyond pancreas
T_4 Tumor involves celiac axis

N_0 No regional lymph nodes
N_1 Regional lymph nodes
N_2 Distant metasis

Treatment

Periampullary–Whipple operation carcinoma body and tail–total pancreatectomy with removal of lymph nodes with radiotherapy 4000–6000 cGy.

QUESTIONS AND ANSWERS

1. **How is pancreatitis diagnosed?**
   Ans: Pancreatitis is likely, in view of the patient's history, namely, recent alcohol abuse followed by development of severe constant epigastric pain that bores through the back, associated nausea and vomiting, and most likely a past history of pancreatitis. The results of his physical examination (tachycardia, hypotension, diaphoresis) is consistent with pancreatitis and hypovolemic shock. Although this patient does not have peritoneal signs, they may be present in severe cases of pancreatitis. One must also entertain other causes of severe epigastric pain, e.g. perforated ulcer, cholecystitis, and mesenteric ischemia.
2. **If present, what is the significance of blue-black discoloration of the patient's flank or periumbilical region?**
   Ans: Through common in acute pancreatitis, both are signs of retroperitoneal hemorrhage and, therefore, hemorrhagic pancreatitis. Ecchymosis of the flank is known as Grey Turner's sign and ecchymosis about the umbilicus known as *Cullen's sign.*
3. **What are Ranson's criteria significance?**
   Ans: Ranson's criteria are a set of indices that statically correlate with an increased risk of death or major complications (Table). These criteria should be evaluated on admission and at 48 hours. The average reported mortality of pancreatitis is 10% but varices according to severity. Patients with 0 to 2 of these criteria have a mortality of 1%; 3 to 4 signs have a 15% mortality; 5 to 6 signs have a 30% mortality, and 7 to 8 signs have a 100% mortality of 1%; 3 to 4 signs have a 15% mortality; 5 to 6 signs have a 30% mortality, and 7 to 8 signs have a 100% mortality. Acute pancreatitis with three or more criteria is considered severe. Serum amylase is not one of Ranson's criteria.

Table: Ranson's criteria

1. Age	>55 years
2. White blood count	>16,000 cells/mm^3
3. Glucose	>200 mg/dl
4. Lactic dehydrogenase	>350 IU/ml
5. Serum alanine aminotransaminase	>250 IU/dl
Signs present during first 48 hours	
6. Hematocrit fall	>10%
7. Blood urea nitrogen rise	>5 mg/dl
8. Calcium	>8 mg/dl
9. Partial pressure oxygen	<60 mm Hg
10. Bas deficit	>4 mEq/L
11. Fluid sequestration	>600 ml

4. What are laboratory changes in acute pancreatitis?
Ans: Hypocalcemia hypoalbuminemia arises from oligenic bone hypovolemia, hypochloremic alkalosis resulting from vomiting, hypovolemia, hyperbilirubinemia, hypoxia may occur. Elevated blood urea nitrogen and creatinine are indicative of hypovolemia, serum amylase level between 200–500 suggests alcoholic etiology.
Serum lipase in better than serum amylase stays elevated for longer time.

5. What are radiological tests for acute pancreatitis?
Ans: Ultrasound, computerized tomography most useful diagnostic tests. Plain X-ray shows perforated viscus dilated, air filled transverse colon. Cut off sign is when gas is not in transverse colon.
CT scan
Grade A : Normal pancreas
Grade B : Pancreas enlargement
Grade C : Grade B and inflammation in peri pancreatic tissue
Grade D : Phlegmon and one fluid collection
Grade E : Phlegmon and two fluid collections.

6. What are complications of acute pancreatitis?
Ans: Hypovolemia with tachycardia, decrease urine output, hypotension, hypocalcemia.

7. What is pseudocyst and treatment?
Ans: Pseudocyst develops in 20% cases of acute pancreatitis, They are unilocular collections of fluid surrounded be fibrous tissue transgastric cystogastrostomy for Psueudocyst adherent to stomach. Gastrojejunostomy with Roux-en-Y loop is for large gut.

8. What are tumor markers with pancreatic cancer?
Ans: CEA and CA 19-9

9. What is treatment based on location
1. Head of pancreas
2. Body of tail
Whipple procedure
Distal resection

10. What is preoperative and postoperative adjuvant therapy?
Ans: Chemotherapy and 5FU

11. What is most common type of pancreatic cancer?
Ans: 90% of pancreatic cancers are ductal cell adenocarcinoma.

12. What radiological investigation for pancreatic cancer?
Ans: Small tumors <2 cm with no local invasion are only pancreatic cancers for resection. Studies are ultrasound, of scan and MRI scan. ERCP can be done to detect duct obstruction.

13. What are signs/symptoms on location?
1. Head of pancreas
Body/tail
Painless jaundice 70%, weight loss 90%, abdominal pain 75%, weakness, pruritis, anorexia, palpable nontender distended gallbladder (Courvoisier sign) alcoholic stools, weight loss and pain 90% migratory thrombophlebitis, jaundice, nausea and vomiting.

Flow Chart: Carcinoma pancreas

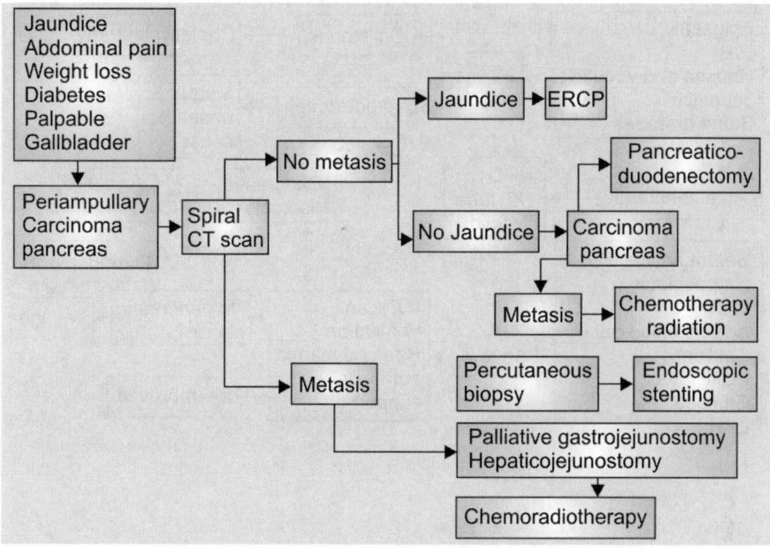

Flow Chart: Pancreatitis

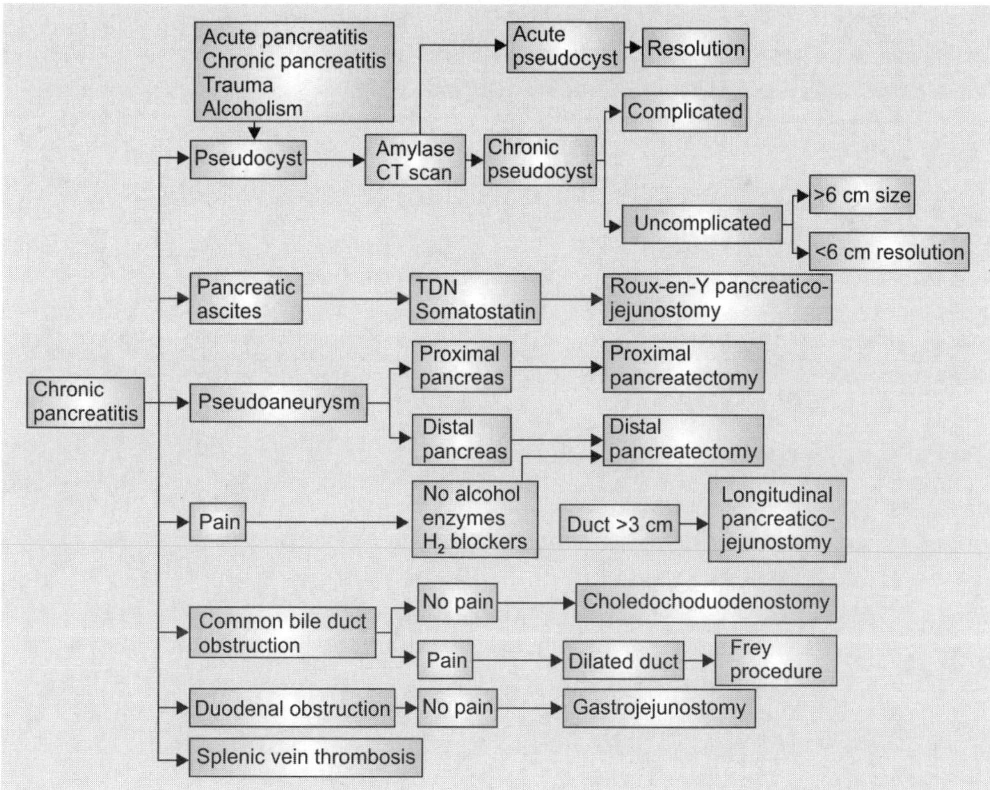

Flow Chart: Pancreatitis

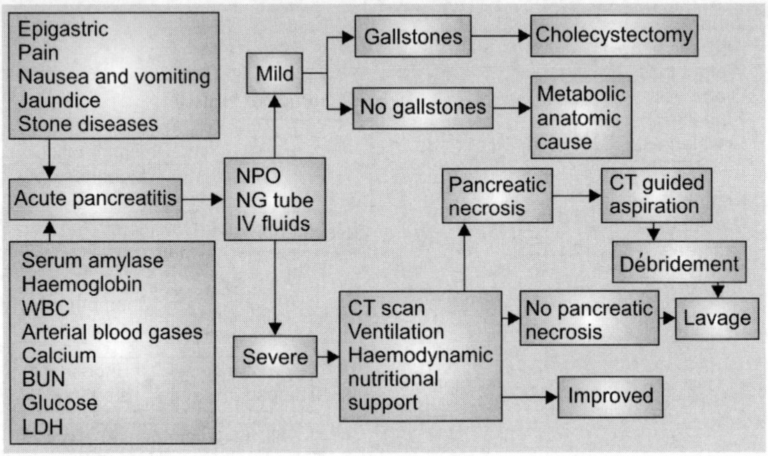

15

Appendix

Caecum and appendix develop from caecal bud arising from postarterial segment of midgut loop.

It arises from posteromedial wall 2 cm below ileocaecal orifice. Length varies from 1–9 inches, diameter–5 mm.

Positions

110 clock–(Paracolic)

12 clock–(Retrocolic or Retrocaecal) 74%

2 clock–(Splenic)

3 clock–Promonteric

4 clock–Pelvic–21%

6 clock–Preileal, postileal

McBurney is site of maximum tenderness junction between lateral 1/3 and medial 2/3 and supplied by appendicular artery which is a branch of ileocolic artery.

Sympathetic nerve supply is T9, 10.

INFLAMMATION OF APPENDIX KNOWN AS APPENDICITIS

Pathophysiology

Obstruction of lumen (Faecolith, extrinsic lymphatic obstruction), bacterial overgrowth and release of activation of local vasoactive peptides, decreased absorptive capacity while mucosa continues to secrete, increased intramural pressure leading to compression of lymphatics, venules, and then arteriolar capillaries which leads to necrosis and perforation.

Diagnosis

1. History–Most common in 2nd or 3rd decade–starts with referred vague visceral pain with periumbilical discomfort, mild nausea, fever, anorexia–pain subsequently localizes to right lower quadrant with local peritoneal irritation and signs.
2. Exam–Tenderness near right lower quadrant (McBurney's point), normal bowel sounds, mild fever, right lower quadrant pain. Hyperaesthesia in right iliac fossa.
   a. Murphy's syndrome–pain, vomiting and fever.
   b. Rovsing's sign–pressure over left iliac fossa causing pain over appendix due to shift of gas toward caecum.

c. Cope psoas test–extension of hip joint produces pain over appendix (Retrocaecal appendix). Retrocaecal appendix may causes haematuria and pain referred to right ureter.
d. Cope's obturator test–patient feels pain where thigh is flexed and medially rotated because obturator internus is stretched. Position test for pelvic appendix.

Treatment

Open appendicectomy–grid, iron, muscle cutting incision at McBurney point and laparoscopic appendectomy.

QUESTIONS AND ANSWERS

1. **What are feature of appendicitis?**
   Ans: Appendicitis present in younger population, second or third decade, pain begins as dull periumbilical discomfort localizing in right lower quadrant.
2. **What is pathophysiology of appendicitis?**
   Ans: Pathophysiology is luminal obstruction caused by lymphoid hyperplasia (60%), faecoliths (35%), foreign bodies (4%), tumour 1%.
3. **How would you manage appendices in pregnancy?**
   Ans: Patients are managed conservatively unless they have appendicular perforation. 2nd Trimester is safe for surgery. How would you manage appendicular with Crohn's disease.
   If base of Appendix and ceacum are not involved in inflammatory process appendectomy is safe.
   How would you manage if you encounter tumor in appendix? Tumor present in appendix is carcinoid 77%. If tumor less than 2 cm then appendectomy is recommended. If tumor >2 cm right hemicolectomy is recommended.
4. **What is blood supply to right colon?**
   Ans: Ileocolic, right colic and middle colic.
5. **Incidence of perforation is greater in what group of patients?**
   Ans: Young children and elderly 75%.
6. **What conditions mimic appendicitis in children?**
   Ans: Mesenteric adenitis.
7. **What described clinical system of appendices?**
   Ans: Fitz in 1886 and tenderness of the right lower quadrant. Recently, *Yersinia enterocolitica* has been identified as a possible cause of both the adenopathy and associated appendicitis.
8. **In which group of patient will the incidence of false-positive diagnosis of appendicitis in chest?**
   Ans: Women between the ages of 20 and 40 years. In common surgical practice it is quite possible to remove appendices that are normal (approximately 15% of all operations). Observation of patients increase both associated morbidity and mortality as a number of perforated appendices increases.

9. **In older patients (age >50 years), what condition may be indistinguishable from acute appendicitis?**
Ans: Acute diverticulitis. Diverticulitis inflammation of either the cecum or a redundant sigmoid may present with right lower quadrant symptoms.
10. **Does in the portal venous system accompanied by chills, fever, and jaundice suggests condition associated with appendicitis?**
*Ans:*Phlebitis, or suppurative thrombosis of the portal vein. Because of preoperative coverage it is now rarely seen after gangrenous or perforated appendicitis.
11. **If the patient explored for right lower quadrant pain has a carcinoma of the caecum, what should the surgeon do?**
Ans: Right hemicolectomy.
12. **What is the most common tumor of the appendix?**
Ans: The carcinoid. It is found in approximately 0.3% of appendectomies.
13. **What is the best treatment of a 2 cm carcinoid involving the best of appendix?**
Ans: Right hemicolectomy.
14. **What is pseudomyxoma peritonei?**
Ans: This term describes the rare laparotomy findings of massive gelatin-like mucinous ascites associated with an ovarian or appendiceal neoplasm. Pseudomyxoma peritonei is perhaps best characterized as a mucin-secreting adenocarcinoma of the ovary or appendix with peritoneal metastasis. The literature is extremely confusing in the differentiation of this condition from benign mucus-producing tumors of the appendix (mucocele) or ovary (cystadenoma). Clinical presentation includes abdominal pain, distention, and small bowel obstruction. Operative intervention is aimed at reduction of tumor bulk. Appendectomy and oophorectomy is advocated. Adjuvant chemotherapy with 5-fluorouracil and melphalan and radiotherapy are of benefit in the postoperative treatment of these patients. Five-year survival is >50%.
15. **Should wide peritoneal drainage be done for treatment of diffuse (perforated) appendiceal peritonitis?**
Ans: No. Wide drainage of the peritoneum has been studied and shown to be unsuccessful and possibly may be harmful to the patient. It is acceptable therapy, however, to mechanically drain loculated intraperitoneal pus (abscess).
16. **Is simple drainage of an appendiceal abscess with appendectomy acceptable treatment of this complication?**
Ans: Yes. In the face of an established abscess with an inaccessible appendix, the abscess is approached and drained mechanically. An appendectomy should be scheduled 6-week later. The incidence of recurrent appendicitis in the un-nerved appendix is approximately 20%.
17. **What is the preferred method of drainage of a pelvis abscess that develops after appendectomy?**
Ans: Transrectal drainage. The approach avoids the peritoneal contamination incurred with transabdominal drainage and should be used if possible.

18. **What is the most common complication following appendectomy?**
Ans: Subcutaneous wound infection.

19. **What is the most common organism of the large bowel in man?**
Ans: Bacteriodes fragilis.

20. **Assuming no antibiotic prophylaxis, what is the frequency of postoperative infections in appendicitis without perforation with perforation?**
Ans: Without perforation, approximately 6–10%. With perforation, approximately 50%.

21. **Has preoperative antibiotic therapy been shown to be of benefit in the management of appendicitis?**
Ans: Yes–In several studies the incidence of infection after appendectomy has been substantially reduced both in perforated and non-perforated cases with administration of a single dose of antibiotic preoperatively.

22. **What is carcinoid tumor?**
Ans: A tumor arising from neuroendocrine cells (APU Domes), Kulchitsky cells.

23. **What is treatment of carcinoid syndrome?**
Ans: Medical therapy is for palliation of carcinoid, syndrome octreatide. somatostatin analogue and cyproheptadine antiserotonin drug. Surgical treatment is excision of primary tumor.

24. **What differential diagnosis of postoperative fever?**
Ans: Wind, water, wound, walk and wonder drugs in first 48 postoperative hours (wind) is most common cause of fever due to lack of deep breathing secondary to pain. Urinary tract infection occurs on 3 to 5 postoperative days. Deep vein thrombosis (walk) can occur with calf tenderness and swelling. Hypersensitivity to drugs causes fever rash.

16

Spleen

ANATOMY

A. Spleen is a lymphatic organ connected to blood vascular system and plans an important role in immune system and acts as filter for blood. It lies in left hypochondruim between 9th and 11th ribs. Spleen is suspended by lineorenal and gastrosplenic ligaments.
B. Usually one lobe but may have lobulations–maintained by four suspensory ligaments.
C. Accessory spleen are congenital mass of splenic tissue with blood supply derived from splenic vessels. Present in 15–30% of patients.
D. Splenosis is bits of splenic tissue embedded in the omentum or mesentery as a result of splenic injury.
E. Histologic architecture involves red pulp (primary vascular) and white pulp (primary lymph tissue) with a portal venous system.
F. Main arterial supply from splenic artery (largest branch of coeliac trunk) but also branch from left gastroepiploic arteries and short gastric artery.
G. Venous drainage includes splenic vein (with numerous pancreatic branches) and short gastric veins. Red pulp has no lymphatics.
H. Pancreas, stomach, adrenal and left kidney can be injured during splenic operations.
I. Sympathetic films derived from coeliac plexus are vasomotor in nature.
J. Develops from cephalic part of dorsal mesogastrium in 6th week of intrauterine life. Blood entering cords and sinuses are open circulation (90%) and blood entering white pulp is closed circulation spleen is palpable of it is enlarged tissue its size.

Function of Spleen

Spleen is suspended by lineorenal and gastrosplenic ligaments

1. Spleen manufacture RBS and WBC in fetus (5th–8th month) until bone marrow matures.
2. Spleen removes pappenheimer siderotic bodies are removed from RBC.
3. Spleen clears blood stream by removing aged red cells by culling.
4. Spleen is reservoir of platelets
5. Spleen secretes antibodies like IgM, tuftin, opsonins, properdin interferons.

Accessory Spleens are Present

- Hilum of spleen
- Splenic vessels
- Tail of pancreas
- Splenic ligaments
- Mesocolon
- Greater omentum.

Splenic Injury

Splenic subscapular haematoma

Patient remains asymptomatic for short period after that haematoma ruptures causing haemorrhage.

Lacerated Wound

Clean incised wounds can be treated by splenorrhaphy. Splenectomy is done for ITP (Idiopathic thrombocytopenic purpura) in which spleen makes antibodies to platelets, hereditary spherocytosis, thalassemias, malignant disease-like staging for Hodgkin's lymphoma.

Primary concern is lack of opsonization of encapsulated bacteria like streptococcus, pneumococcus, pneumococcus lowering sepsis and death. Pneumococcal vaccine is given preoperatively.

Penicillin prophylaxis should be splenectomy given. Splenic cysts are treated with splenectomy.

It is done through midline/subcostal incision. After incision ligaments of spleen splenic artery, vein and short gastric vessels are ligated.

Partial Splenectomy

It can be done by retaining upper or lower polar branches of splenic artery.

Splenorrhaphy

Spleen can be salvaged by suturing wound by placing gelfoam and thrombin. Laparoscopic splenectomy with or without hand port is becoming treatment of choice in patients of haematological disorders like ITP and hereditary spherocytes having smaller spleens.

QUESTIONS AND ANSWERS

1. **Which intra-abdominal organs are injured most frequently, and which would you suspect are injured in this patients?**

   Ans: The most frequently injured organs are, in descending order, spleen (26.2%), kidneys (24.2%), intestines (16.2%), and liver (15.6%). Considering the location, the most likely injury, if any, would be that of the spleen.

2. **What physical signs would expect in the presence of splenic injury?**
Ans: Left upper quadrant abdominal pain in present in only 33% of all splenic injuries, and of all ruptured spleen, only 50 to 60% manifest tender abdomen with guarding and distension, and of all ruptured (systolic blood pressure <100 mm Hg) is present in only 30 to 40% cases.
3. **What are physical signs associated with splenic injury?**
Ans: Splenic Injury: **(1) Balance's sign:** Dullness to percussion in the left flank and a shifting dullness in the right flank. **(2) Kehr's sign:** left shoulder pain as a result of irritation of the inferior surface of the left hemidiaphragm by blood clots.
4. **What is Kehr's sign?**
Ans: Left shoulder pain with splenic rupture.
5. **What is balance sign?**
Ans: LUQ dullness to percussion.
6. **How is spleen injury diagnosed?**
Ans: Abdominal ultrasound, CT scan is it patient is stable.
7. **What is splenorrhaphy?**
Ans: Splenic salvage operation, wrapping mesh or partial splenectomy.
8. **What are investigations for splenic injury?**
Ans: Diagnostic peritoneal lavage (DPL), CT scan, ultrasound and radionuclide scanning.
9. **Describe anatomy of spleen**
Ans: Spleen lies in left upper quadrant posterolaterally between 9th to 11th ribs. It is held by suspensary ligaments splenorenal, splenophrenic and splenocolic. The arterial supply is from splenic artery and short gastric artery.
10. **Describe embryology of spleen**
Ans: Spleen develops in 5th week of gestation when mesenchymal cells fuse to from spleen.
11. **What happen after splenectomy?**
Ans: There is impaired phagocytic activity to incapsulated bacterial organisms, decreased level of globulin, decreased T cell function, decreased opsonication, and decreased properdin levels.
12. **In what splenic injury would splenic preservation be indicated?**
Ans: In nonbleeding capsular lacerations spleen should be left packing should be applied to minor lacerations. Parenychymal tears are to suture ligations. Extensive parenchymal tears not in vicinity of can be treated with partial splenectomy.
13. **What are steps for splenectomy?**
Ans: Suspensory ligaments are divided and spleen is dissected anteromedially along the hilum and pancreas. Visualize the posterior aspect of splenic pedicle. Hilar vessels should be ligated. When mobilizing spleen greater curvature of stomach must be left intact to prevent gastric fistulas.
14. **Arterial supply of spleen**
Ans: Splenic artery branch of celiac trunk and short gastric arise from gastroepiploic arteries.
15. **What is venous drainage of spleen?**
Ans: Portal vein via splenic vein and left gastroepiploic vein.

16. **What are functions of spleen?**
Ans: It filters abnormal, RBC, stores platelets produces opsonines, produces antibodies and site of phagocytosis.
17. **What parentage of total platelets stored in spleen?**
Ans: 33%
18. **What are functions of spleen?**
Ans: It filters RBC, stores platelets, produces tuftsin and properdin, produces antibodies and site of phagocytosis.
19. **Commonest intra-abdominal organ injured during blunt trauma.**
Ans: Spleen
20. **What is delayed splenic rupture?**
Ans: Subcapsular haematoma may rupture any time after blunt trauma occurs after 2 weeks after injury present with shock and abdominal pain.
21. **What are signs of ruptured spleen?**
Ans: Haemoperitoneum and Kehr sign, LUQ abdominal pain and Ballance sign.
22. **What are indications of splenectomy?**
Ans: Hodgkin staging, splenic tumors, hypersplenism, medullary fibrosis, hereditary elliptocytosis, sickle cell anemia, ITP, haemolytic anaemia, heriditary spherocytosis and thalassemias.

17

Small Bowel

ANATOMY

Duodenum: C-shaped tube lying in front of and right of inferior vena cava and aorta.

1st 2.5 cm contained between peritoneum of lesser and greater omentum and divided into:

First part of superior which is 2" long, ascends from gastroduodenal junction and anterior to portal vein and CBD and gastroduodenal artery.

Second part is 3" long and anterior is gallbladder, transverse colon, small gut, postoperative is renal vessels, pelvis, right is hepatic flexure of colon and left is head of pancreas.

Third part is 4" long, anterior is superior mesenteric vessels, root of mesentery, transverse colon and mesocolon, posterior is inferior vena cava, spermatic vessels, left sympathetic trunk and left psoas muscle, superior is head of pancreas and inferior is small gut.

Blood supply–superior pancreaticoduodenal artery branch of gastroduodenal artery and inferior pancreaticoduodenal first branch of superior mesenteric artery.

Jejunum–central 2/3 of small bowel

Ileum–distal 1/3 of small bowel.

From duodenal-jejunal junction to mid-transverse colon blood supply is from superior mesenteric artery and vein.

They have Peyer's patches, ileocaecal valve and occasionally meckel diverticulum (which is within 2 feet of ileocaecal valve, antimesenteric border, point of intussusception in 2 year old, in 2% of population and 2" in length.

Peritoneum is divided into visceral which surrounds the viscera and parietal which lies the rest of cavity. Parietal is painful and supplied by somatic nerves and visceral is poorly supplies by nerves and pain is poorly localized.

Greater omentum is abdominal policeman attached to greater curvature of stomach and lesser omentum is attached to lesser curvature of stomach. Greater omentum is pushed by movement into area of immobility where there is local peritoneal irrigation.

Mesenteric attachment runs from left to right duodenojejunal flexure of L3 to right sacroiliac joint.

Mesentery of judgment has only two series of arcades where as lower ileum has several arcades.

Large intestine can be distinguished from small intestine by presence of *Taenia coli* and appendices epiploicae. Small bowel has conniventes that completely cross the lumen and large bowel has haustral folds which do not cross all the lumen's width.

PHYSIOLOGY

Absorption/Digestion

1. Break down of proteins to polypeptides, fats to fatty acids and complex carbohydrates (CHO) to simple sugars begins in duodenum with various enzymes (trypsin, chymotrypsin, elastase, lipase, amylase.
2. Absorption occurs in bowel–proteins and CHO by active processes and lipids by passive diffusion.
3. Ileum–specialized absorption of iron (with intrinsic factor secreted by stomach), lipids and bile salts (enterohepatic circulation).

Motility

1. Parasympathetic innervations from vagus (X), increased tone and intestinal motility.
2. Intrinsic motility is present in response to changes in intraluminal pressures.
3. Sympathetics innervations slows tone and motility.

Endocrine

1. Multiple hormones including VIP, secretin and enterogastrone.
2. Trophic hormones for bowel mucosa growth.

Crohn's Disease

Regional enteritis is granulomatous, non-caseating inflammatory condition of ileum and colon.

Most Common Enteritis Disease of Small Bowel

1. Etiology unknown
2. Increased incidence 2nd–3rd decade and 6th–7th decade
3. Non-caseating granulomatous inflammation of entire bowel wall
4. Skip areas frequent–fissures in mucosa
5. Most commonly involves terminal ileum; can involve any part of the bowel
6. May cause enteral fistulae and transmural inflammation.

Manifestations

1. Crampy abdominal pain, low grade fever, bloody diarrhea and weight loss
2. May present like acute appendicitis
3. May present with persistent perianal disease–fistula, fissures and abscesses.

Diagnosis

1. Barium enema, UGI with small bowel follow through–"string" sign in distal ileum

2. Colonoscopy if within reach of the instruments–cobblestone, linear erosions/ fissures and thickening of bowel. Hose pipe appearance straightening of valvulae conniventes.

Treatment

1. Azulfidine/prednisone for acute flare-ups. May need parenteral hyperalimentation
2. Maintenance medication occasionally helpful azothioprine, salazopyrine.
3. Surgical excision for:
   a. Haemorrhage
   b. Obstruction
   c. Perforation
   d. Intractable symptoms
   e. Recurrence rate of approximately 50% in 8 years.

Surgical treatment is strictures treated by stricture plasty perforations require resection. Pancolic disease requires total proctocolectomy and ileostomy.

Small Bowel Obstruction

Etiology

1. Postoperative adhesions (60%)
2. Incarceration in hernias (20%)
3. Others–Crohn's intussusception, volvulus and tumors.

Types of Obstruction

1. Simple obstruction–most common, vomiting, abdominal and distention
2. Closed loop obstruction–early necrosis and perforation with minimal prodromal illness (i.e, volvulus, etc.)
3. Partial obstruction–continues to pass gas and occasionally will resolve spontaneously
4. Strangulated obstruction–bowel necrosis.

Diagnosis

1. History–nausea, vomiting, obstipation, crampy abdominal pain
2. Physical exam–distended, tympanic abdomen and hyperactive pain
3. X-ray–dilated loops small bowel, air-fluid level and no gas in colon.

Treatment

1. Fluid resuscitation
2. Correct isotonic fluid losses plus hypokalemic, hypochloremic metabolic alkalosis
3. NG decompression
4. Early laparotomy to relieve the obstruction, resection and end-to-end anastomosis.

Differential Diagnosis

	Paralytic ileus	*Small intestinal obstruction*
1.	Minimal abdominal pain	Crampy abdominal pain
2.	Nausea and vomiting	Nausea and vomiting
3.	Obstruction and failure to pass flatus	Obstipation and failure to pass flatus
4.	Abdominal distention	Abdominal distention
5.	Decreased or absent bowel sounds	Normal or increased bowel sounds
6.	Gas in small intestinal and colon on X-ray	Gas in the small intestine only on X-ray

Look for abnormal quantity of gas in stomach, small intestine or colon normal diameter 2.5 cm small, 5 cm colon and 7 cm caecum.

In small bowel obstruction vomiting occurs earlier, distention is less and pain is higher in abdomen.

X-ray shows central gas shadows and no gas in large bowel.

Obstruction in mechanical GI obstruction where no cause found treat conservatively congenital hypertrophic stenosis present in 1st 3–8 weeks. Projectile vomiting, malnourished, mass could be felt. Treatment is elaborate correction and Ramsted pyloromyotomy.

Interruption

Episodic inconsolable crying in 5–12 months with drawing the legs up colic and vomiting. Sausage shaped abdominal mass plain X-ray, ultrasound and CT scan. Laparotomy and excision of necrotic bowel.

Peritonitis

Perforation of peptic ulcer, diverticulum, appendix, bowel of gas bladder, signs are prostration, shock rebound tenderness, board like rigidity. Except X-Ray, shows gas under diaphragm. Necessitates laparotomy.

In diverticulum, cholecystitis, salphingitis and appendicitis. If abscess forms swelling ultrasound guided aspiration and laparotomy.

Small Bowel Cancers

Benign tumors include polyps, leiomyomas, symptomatic lesions are resected.

Adenocarcinoma most common and intrinsic cancer of small bowel (most common in jejunum).

1. Carcinoids in small bowel, second only to appendix
   a. Carcinoid syndrome–associated with liver metasis–consists of episodes of serotonin surge, flushing hyperperistalsis, diarrhoea, bronchospasm, etc. (5 HT)
2. Lymphoma also may involve small bowel
3. Occasionally leiomyosarcoma
   Signs/Syndrome–primarily obstruction and occasional bleeding.

Treatment of Most Tumours Revolves Around Excision

1. Lymphoma is responsive to chemotherapy
   Acute small bowel ischemia may follow superior mesenteric artery embolism or thrombosis, low flow states or venous thrombosis, is commonest cause.
   Treat severe abdominal pain, hypovolaemia, raised plasma amylase and metabolic acidosis. Treatment is fluid replacement, antibiotics and heparin, surgery includes resection should be done and tumour of small intestine removed.

QUESTIONS AND ANSWERS

1. **Why is testing the stool for blood important?**
   Ans: Haem-positive stool may be an early indication of ischemia bowel. The muscosa of the bowel wall is most susceptible to ischemia and will slough before full thick injury occurs. The bowel is still viable if full thickness necrosis has not occurred. Also, haem-positive stool increased the likelihood of a cancerous etiology for obstruction in this patient with previous colon cancer.
2. **What is the significance of the quality of the bowel sounds?**
   Ans: In the early period of obstruction, peristalsis is increased and hyperactive bowel sounds occur in rushes in an attempt to overcome the obstruction. As the bowel distends, reflux inhibition of bowel motility can result in a quiet abdomen. The quality of the bowel sounds does not help in differentiating between a partial and complete obstruction.
3. **What is anatomy of small intestine?**
   Ans: duodenum, jejunum, ileum comprises small intestine, Length is 6 meter (20 feet). Duodenum is 12 inches. Blood supply is superior mesenteric artery. Circular folds of mucosa plicae are present in lumen. Jejunum–large plicae circular, thicker. Ileum–smaller plicae, thinner.
4. **What is small intestinal obstruction?**
   Ans: Mechanical obstruction to passage of intraluminal contents. Clinical features are pain, distention, hypochloremic hypokalemia, hernias, X-ray shows distended loops and air fluid levels on up right X-rays, CT scan and barium follow through are done.
5. **What are causes of small bowel obstruction?**
   Ans: Adhesions, bulge, cancer and tumors acronym Gives Bad Cramps
   G Gallstone ileus
   I Intussusception
   V Volvulus
   E External compression
   S SMA syndrome
   B Bezoars
   A Abscess
   D Diverticulitis
   C Crohn's disease
   R Radiation enteritis
   A Annular pancreas
   M Meckel's diverticulum
   P Peritoneal adhesions
   S Stricture
6. **What are benign and malignant tumors of small intestine?**
   Ans: Leiomyomas common benign small intestinal tumor.

Adenocarcinoma commonest malignant small intestinal tumor. Other causes are carcinoid 25%, lymphoma (20%) sarcomas.

7. **What is Meckel's diverticulum?**
Ans: Remnant of omphalomesenteric duct 2 feet from ileocaecal junction, 2% population, symptoms are haemorrhage, obstruction and inflammation. Treatment is surgical resection. Meckel's hernia is called Littre hernia.
8. **What is commonest cause of small intestine bleeding?**
Ans: Small intestine angiodysplasias.
9. **What are operations of obstruction of small bowel?**
Ans: Lysis of adhesions, resection of obstructed lesions in small intestine, reduction and repair of hernias.
10. **What is tracheoesophageal fistula?**
Ans: Esophageal atresia and fistula at distal pouch
Esophageal atresia and fistula at proximal pouch
Tracheoesophageal fistula without atresia H-type.
Diagnosis is made by inability to pass nasogastric tube beyond 12 cm. Treatment is esophageal anastomosis.
11. **What is common diaphragmatic hernia?**
Ans: Posterolateral foramen of Bochdalek infants present with respiratory distress, dyspnea, X-ray shows air-filled intestine.
12. **What is intussusception?**
Ans: 90% idiopathic, ileocolic, colo-colic, intussusceptum. Outer part is intussuscipients child complaints of abdominal pain. Treatment is surgery.

Flow Chart: Small bowel obstruction

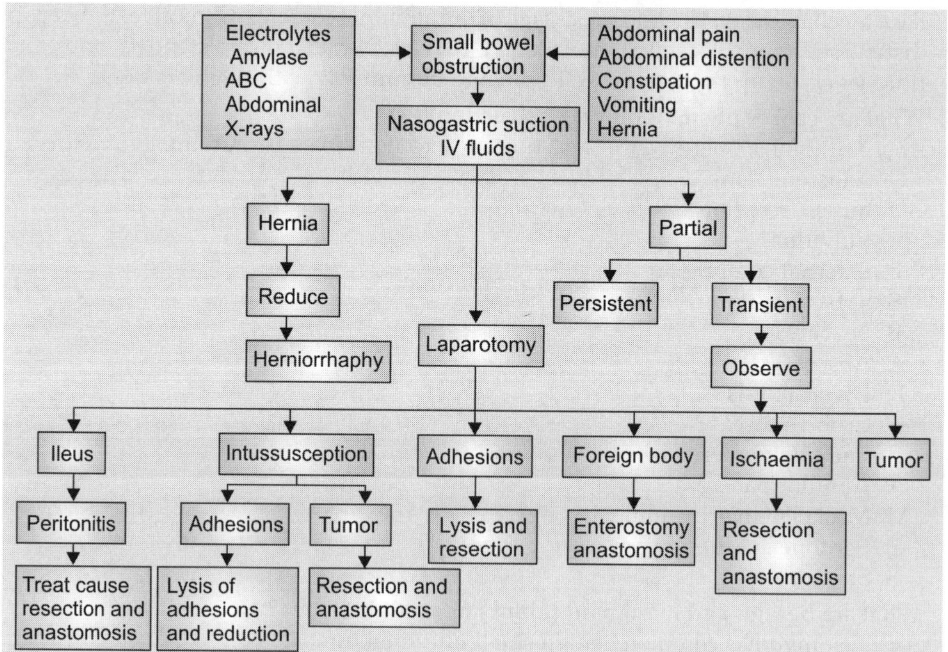

Flow Chart: Upper abdominal pain

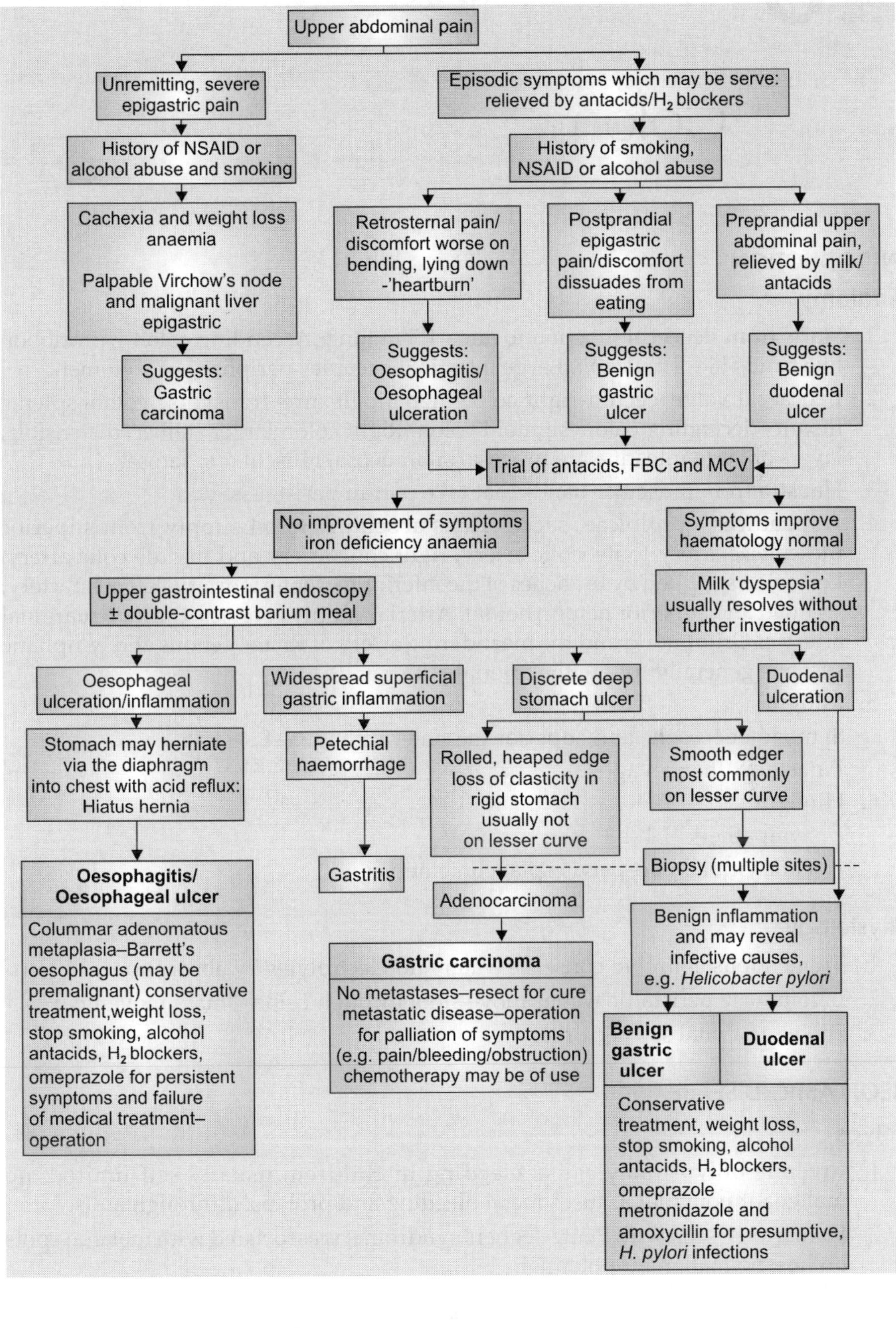

18

Colon

INTRODUCTION

Anatomy

1. Starts from ileocecal junction to anus 1.5 m long. Ascending colon with ribbon like bands like *Taenia coli*. Large intestinal occupies periphery of abdomen.
2. Ileocaecal valve–cecum-right colon–hepatic flexure–transverse colon–splenic flexure–decending colon–sigmoid colon. Right colon larger caliber, distensible, layers of large intestine are mucosa, submucosa, muscular's, serosa.
3. Haustra from muscular bands that take part in peristalsis.
4. Appendices, epiploicae, sacculations absent. Arterial supply from superior mesenteric artery to ileocolic artery, right colic artery and middle colic artery. Left colon supplied by branches of the inferior mesenteric artery–left colic artery, sigmoid and superior hemorrhoidal. Arterial supply connects through marginal artery of Drummond and the meandering artery of Rilan. Venous and lymphatic systems generally follow the arterial patterns.
5. Midgut
   Sympathetic–coelic and superior mesenteric ganglia–T11- L1
   Parasympathetic–vagus
6. Hindgut
   Sympathetic–L1–L3
   Parasympathetic–pelvic splanchnic nerves.

Physiology

1. Tremendous ability to conserve water and electrolytes by absorption
2. Involuntary peristaltic waves move stool through colon–"mass movement"
3. Serves as a vital storage organ.

NEOPLASTIC DISEASE

Polyps

1. Juvenile polyps–may cause bleeding in children; usually self-limited; no malignant potential. Causes rectal bleeding and prolapsed through anus.
2. Hamartous–seen with Peutz-Jeghers syndrome; is associated with melanin spots on lips; no malignant potential.

3. Tubular adenomas–most common types of polyps found; usually small (<0.5 cm); low malignant potential (5% associated with cancers) unless numerous or large (>1 cm).
   a. Familial polyposis: Autosomal dominant disease of thousands of tubular adenomatous polyps in colon; usually colon removed prophylactically (usually done as total abdominal colectomy, rectal mucosectomy, ileoanal pouch anastomosis to certain continence). (0.5 to 5 cm).
   b. Gardener syndrome: Autosomal dominant–tubular adenomatous throughout GI tract (although not as numerous as familial polyposis); associated with exostosis (esp. Maxilla) and inclusion cysts in skin.
   c. Villotubular adenomas: Histologic picture of both tubular and villous elements; less common than tubular adenomas but higher association with malignancy (approximately 20%).
   d. Villous adenomas–10% of all benign lesions of colon, single, papillary, more unusual than villotubular adenomas but higher malignant potential (approximately 35%) especially if larger (>3 cm). May cause a syndrome of watery diarrhea with huge loses of KCl resulting in hypokalemia.
   e. Turcot's: Autosomal recessive, colonic polyps and neurological tumours.
4. Adenocarcinoma of colon
   a. Most common visceral cancer in United States–behind only lung and breast as cause of cancer deaths.
   b. Etiology unknown thought to be related to dietary habits high in animal fats and low in fibre. Higher association with various polyps, ulcerative colitis, Crohn's colitis and lymphogranuloma venarum, higher socioeconomic status.
   c. More common in left and sigmoid colon (50%–70%).
      - Synchronous tumours in 5%
      - Metachronous tumours 3–5%
5. Left side tumors tend to develop into constricting "apple-core" lesions, circumferential resulting in symptoms of " constipation", pencil-thin stools, occult blood with abdominal pain in (50–70%), change in bowel habit (60%), palpable mass (45%) occasional bright red blood, partial or total bowel obstruction.
6. Right sided tumours tend to develop into polypoid, ulcerating, fungating masses which cause anemia resulting in fatigue, weight loss, poor appetite, occult blood in stool, abdominal pain (80%), abdominal mass (67%) and weight loss (48%).
7. Both are diagnosed by colonoscopy with biopsy or barium enema. 5% incidence of synchronous lesions (other tumors present at the same time but different place). Filling defect with typical finger print deformity or shouldering, tumor maker are CEA.
8. Prognosis is most related to lymphatic involvement and metastatic spread various modification of Duke's classification scheme are used.
   a. Disease limited to mucosa, 80–90% 5-year survival. (Stage-A)
   b. Disease through wall of colon, no lymph node or distant spread, 60–70% 5-year survival. (Stage-B_1)

9. Disease involves lymph nodes limited to wall, 30% 5-year survival. (Stage-C_1)
10. Lesions involving all layers, Distant metastases, <5% 5-year survival (Stage-C_2).
11. TNM Classification
    - T_x Primary tumour cannot be assessed
    - T_0 No evidence of primary tumour
    - T_1 CA *in situ* or invasion of lamina propria
    - T_2 Tumour invades propria
    - T_3 Tumour invades subserosa
    - T_4 Invades other organs
    - N_x Regional lymph nodes cannot be assessed
    - N_o No regional lymph nodes
    - N_1 Metastasis to 1–3 regionally lymph nodes
    - N_2 Metastasis to 4 or more regional lymph nodes
    - M_1 Presence of metastasis.
12. Treatment involves removal of tumor bearing colon, along with wide margins of normal colon and the lymphatic drainage bed. Local excision is possible in T_1 and T_3 lesion within 6 cm of anal verge in well and moderate differentiated lesions with no vascular or lymphatic extensions. Radiotherapy for palliation.
    a. CA caecum or ascending colon is treated by right hemicolectomy
    b. CA hepatic flexure is–extended right hemicolectomy
    c. CA transverse colon–extended right hemicolectomy
    d. CA splenic flexure–anterior resection
    e. CA pelvic colon–extended left hemicolectomy
    f. Hepatic metasis are treated with cytotoxic drugs or by-pass procedure
    g. Hepatic metasis are treated with cytotoxic drugs or cryo or laser surgery.
    i. Laparoscopic colon–Rectal surgery has achieved equal results to open resection in terms of long-term survival, resonance rates and wound metasis.
13. Isolated metastases to liver can be removed with improved long-term survival.
14. Various large-scale screening efforts to detect the cancer earlier (including proctoscopy, feacal occult blood testing, CEA antigen levels in serum).
15. Chemotherapy for metastatic disease has had limited success; radiation therapy has not been helpful except in reducing the bulk of large rectal cancers.

INFLAMMATORY DISEASES

Diverticulitis

1. Diverticulitis remucosal hernias through the muscularis and occur at points in the colon where end arteries enter the bowel wall; are thought to be related to diets low in fibre/bulk–they occur in most people in Western cultures who lives long enough–present in up to 70% of elderly patients, more common in left colon. Colonic mucosal protrudes through circular muscle, occur in rows mostly found in sigmoid colon, saw tooth appearance in ba-enema.

2. Erosion into an adjacent artery, without inflammation, may lead to massive blood loss (diverticulosis).
3. Obstruction of the lumen of a diverticulum leads to bacterial overgrowth, swelling, inflammation and possibly to rupture and abscess formation– "diverticulum". Inflammation of one diverticulitis or more over the age of 40.
4. Presentation is like a "left-sided" appendicitis in older patients causes heaviness, distention and flatulence.
5. Treatment of mild cases involves antibiotics against coliforms, high bulk, high fibre diet, hydration. Cases involving intractable symptoms or repeated episodes, hemorrhage, obstruction due to stricture formation or perforation may need surgical removal of the diseased colon. One stage operation with removal of affected segment and end-to-end anastomosis.
6. Diverticular disease of colon.

PATHOGENESIS

Low fibre diet
↓
Inappropriate segmentation of colonic circular muscle
↓
'segmental intraluminal hypertension'
↓
Gross thickening of circular muscle
Pulsion diverticulae

Treatment of Uncomplicated Diverticular Disease

High residue diet: Fresh fruit and vegetables
Whole meal bread and flour
Unprocessed bran
Bulk purgatives

Antispasmodics: Intraluminal colonic pressure is abnormally high in diverticular disease, and gastrointestinal transit time is prolonged. Unprocessed bran lowers intraluminal pressure and shortens transit time

Complication of Diverticular Disease

1. Diverticulitis: Localised peritonitis
Generalised peritonitis
2. Haemorrhage
3. Colonic stenosis and obstruction
4. Fistula formation: Vesicocolic
Enterocolic
Colo-colic
Colo-vaginal
5. Small bowel intestinal obstruction

Indication for Surgery

1. Severe progressive inflammatory disease (Recurrent episodes of acute diverticulitis).
2. Failure to control long standing symptoms by medical means
3. Colonic strictures and the possibility of malignancy
4. General peritonitis
5. Massive, continuous, uncontrolled haemorrhage
6. Fistulae

Treatment of Complication of Diverticular Disease

1. Acute diverticulitis with localized peritonitis
   Intravenous fluids
   Antibiotics
2. Acute diverticulitis with generalized peritonitis
   Intensive treatment of fluid depletion and shock (hypovolaemic or bacteraemic) in preparation of surgery
   i. Purulent turbid peritonitis (rupture of pericolic abscess)
      a. Peritoneal toilet
      b. Pelvic drain
      c. Antibiotics
      d. Management of ileus
   ii. Faecal peritonitis
      a. Resection of inflamed bowel without primary anastomosis
         Mikulicz resection
         Hartmann resection
         Restoration of colonic continuity at a secondary procedure
      b. Defunctioning colostomy and pelvic drainage
         An alternative if resection is not technically possible
3. Massive, continuous, uncontrolled haemorrhage
   In many series reviewing haemorrhage in diverticular disease, the source of the bleeding in more than half the cases occurred in the ascending or proximal transverse colon
   i. Total colectomy with ileostomy or ileorectal haemorrhage
   ii. Subtotal colectomy with caecoproctostomy
   iii. Conservative resection following accurate localization of bleeding site by selective arteriography
4. Ulcerative colitis
   i. Inflammatory process of colonic mucosa and submucosa of unknown etiology; usually appears in 2nd–3rd decade, but a second peak incidence around age 55.
      a. Mucosal immunological reaction
      b. Weakened mucosal reaction
      c. Defective mucosal barrier metabolism

ii. Signs and symptoms–crampy abdominal pain, bloody mucous diarrhea often fever, weight loss, fatigue, etc. Clinical picture varies from (55% of patients) to acute fulminant illness with massive dilatation of colon and sepsis (15% of patients) (toxic megacolon). Process is repeated episodes of illness with cramps, bloody diarrhea and associated symptoms. 90% disease start in rectum and spreads proximally and involves till 30 cm of ileum.
iii. Diagnosis is usually with colonoscopy (erosion of mucosa with "pseudopolyps) covers large areas, no skip areas or barium enema during quiescent phases (foreshortening of colon, loss of haustra, "lead pipe" (appearance), narrow contractive colon.
iv. Symptoms can often be controlled (80%) with systemic steroids, azulfidine and motility inhibitors (codeine) steroids with prednisolone (20–40 mg per day), sulphasalazine 1 gm t.d.s.
v. Long-term risk includes increased risk of cancer–4% at 10 years and cancer risk increased by approximately 2% per year thereafter. Greater amount colon involved and greater activity of the disease leads to even greater cancer risk.
vi. Disease is cured by removal of all colon mucosa–usually done as total colectomy, rectal mucosectomy, ileoanal reservoir anastomosis. Permanent proctocolectomy and ileostomy, restorative proctocolectomy with ileoanal pouch (PARK), colectomy with ileorectal anastomosis, ileostomy with intra-abdominal pouch.

CROHN'S DISEASE

Chronic inflammatory disease of ileum and ileocolonic disease is commonest presentation 60% ileal and 30% large intestine.

Narrowing lumen, deep mucosal ulceration, cobblestone appearance, mesenteric abscesses. Earliest mucosal lesions are discrete aphthous ulcers. Symptoms resemble acute appendicitis. Investigation are colonoscopy which allow irregular length of terminal ileum involved–string sign of kantor.

Medical Treatment of Crohn's Disease

1. Salazopyrine
2. Steroids
3. Azathioprine
   a. Active disease not responding to steroids alone and where surgery is contra-indicated
   b. Fistulae–some will improve or heal
   c. Peri-operatively to reduce suture line recurrence, dehiscence and fistula formation
4. Correction of anaemia
5. Correction of hypoproteinaemia
   a. Will improve as inflammation is suppressed
   b. Parenteral alimentation is suppressed

6. Control of diarrhea
   a. Low fat diet if steatorrhoea is a feature
   b. Codeine, lomotil
   c. Cholestyramine: Bile salts not absorbed by ileum have cathartic action on colon.

Indications for Surgery

1. Abscess
2. Fistulae
3. Stricture
4. Perforation
5. Obstruction
6. Failure to suppress active disease medical means where the disease is not so extensive that surgery is contraindicated and where an operative mortality of approximately 3% is acceptable.
7. Uveitis, recurrent polyarthritis and pyoderma gangrenosa.

Surgical Management of Crohn's Disease

1. Drainage of abscess
   In chronic disease
   Continuous symptoms
   Recurrent polyarthritis
   Fibrous strictures
   Carcinomas or the risk of developing carcinoma.

Surgical Treatment

In acute attack

1. Transverse colostomy: In fulminating case where the patient is too ill for colectomy.
2. Colectomy, ileostomy and rectosigmoid fistula.
   a. With later conversion to ileorectal anastomosis.

In chronic attack

1. Colectomy with ileorectal anastomosis with or without a temporary ileostomy
2. Subtotal colectomy with caecoproctomy
3. Panproctocolectomy and ileostomy.

Complications of Surgery

General:	Haemorrhage	
	Pulmonary infection and collapse	
	Wound sepsis	
	DVT, pulmonary embolism	
Specific:	Peritonitis	Localised
		Septicaemic shock

Adhesions to bare colonic bed
Adhesions to pelvic floor
Internal hernia through paraileostomy space
Ileostomy prolapsed, regression or stenosis
Perineal status
Skin excoriation related to ileostomy
Paraileostomy hernia
Retraction of rectosigmoid mucous fistula.

LARGE BOWEL OBSTRUCTION

A. Colon cancer (65%)
B. Diverticular disease (20%)
Symptoms are pain suprapubic, vomiting, abdominal distention, diarrhoea, constipation and fever, mass left lower abdomen. X-ray shows distended colon with typical haustral markings, absence of air in rectum.
C. Volvulus (5%)–sigmoid followed by a caecum–more common in older patients, poor colonic function–long mesentery which allow twisting of the involved segment. Diagnosis with plain X-rays of abdomen. Sigmoid volvulus occasionally relieved with rectal tube but often recurs, requiring removal of sigmoid. Caecal volvulus usually treated with caecopexy if bowel wall viability not in question.
D. Tuberculosis of large intestine could be hyperplastic with intestinal obstruction treatment is ATT and resection in cases of obstruction.
E. Pseudo-obstruction–(Ogilvie's syndrome) dilated portion of colon–usually transverse and right side without mechanical lesion; usually in older patients often on digoxin and anti-Parkinson medication.
F. Treatment of colon obstruction usually requires colostomy and removal of offending portion with reanastomosis done separately after the colon can be prepared.

LOWER GI HEMORRHAGE

A. Melaena
1. Source can be anywhere in GI tract–requires only approximately 50 cc blood to create guaiac positive stools.
2. Most common source of melaena is UGI bleed, therefore investigate esophagus, stomach, duodenum and get endoscopy.
3. Sources below ligament of Treitz include small bowel tumors (polyps or cancers), Meckel's diverticulum, Crohn's disease, AV malformations, diverticulosis and ulcerative colitis.
4. Management includes fluid resuscitation, restoration of clotting factors and search for etiology.
5. Colonoscopy and arteriography are most useful diagnostic tools. Labelled RBC nuclear scans are occasionally helpful.
6. Surgical exploration without a diagnosis or location of bleeding preoperatively is often unrewarding.

B. Hematochezia: Bright red blood per rectum
   1. Consider diverticulosis, colonic telangiectasis (AV malformations), hemorrhoids, colon cancers
   2. May occasionally occur with massive upper GI bleed
   3. Colostomy is an artificial opening made in large bowel to divert faeces and flatus to exterior.
      Temporary, double barreled and permanent
      Complication: Necrosis, lateral space obstruction, stenosis, herniation and prolapsed.

QUESTION AND ANSWERS

1. **Where are the most common areas of colorectal recurrence?**
   Ans: Local recurrence and regional lymph node invasion are the most common, followed by metastases to liver, followed by lung and bone.
2. **What is familial adenomatous polyposis (FAP)? How is it related to colorectal carcinoma?**
   Ans: FAP is an autosomal dominant hereditary disease in which adenomatous polyps carpet the large intestine, usually beginning around adolescence. These polyps have a tendency to undergo malignant transformation.
3. **What causes colonic diverticula?**
   Ans: Colonic diverticular are outpouchings of mucosa, submucosa, and muscularis mucosa through the muscular wall of the colon. Their formation may be related to either weakness of the bowel wall at sites of vessel performation or to increased intraluminal pressure caused by low dietary fibre and constipation.
4. **Where are diverticula usually located in the colon?**
   Ans: Most are in the left colon, but diverticula of the right colon and caecum are not rare.
5. **At what age is diverticulitis most common?**
   Ans: After age 50: Approximately 5–10% of patients are under age 40. These patients frequently require operative treatment.
6. **What procedure is required to repair vesicocolic or ureterocolic fistula?**
   Ans: If pneumaturia occurs early after diverticulitis, a proximal diverting colostomy is performed. About 3 months later, the involved colon is resected, the colostomy is taken down, and the colon. About 3 months later, the involved colon is resected, the colostomy is taken down, and the colon is anastomosed primarily. If pneumaturia occurs late or is longstanding, preliminary diversion by means of colostomy is unnecessary.
7. **How is the diagnosis confirmed?**
   Ans: Patient will complain of nausea, vomiting, distention, and obstruction. Vomiting in a distal obstruction occurs later and may be feculent in nature. Physical examination reveals distention and high-pitched bowel sounds with rashes. These symptoms can progress to silence and localized tenderness, which are serious signs.
   Plain abdominal films reveal gas in the dilated colon with haustral markings. An upright chest film may show free air under the diaphragm if a perforation has occurred.
8. **How is the diagnosis confirmed?**
   Ans: Plain abdominal films are usually sufficient to conform a diagnosis. However, barium enema is confirmatory and can further delineate the level and nature of an obstruction. A stricture can also be demonstrated with the use of a contrast enema.

9. **What causes large bowel obstruction?**
Ans: Mechanical: Carcinoma (50–70%), volvulus (15–25%), diverticular disease (5–10%). Non-mechanical: Neuromuscular disorders such as toxic megacolon and paralytic ileus (Ogilvie's syndrome).
10. **Which operation should be performed?**
Ans: It is important to decompress the colon before it perforates; therefore, the standard procedure is a decomposing colostomy. Adequate resection of a malignant tumour cannot be done satisfactorily under emergency conditions. Diverticular disease can be resected; however, an anastomosis can be done primarily because of the presence of infection. Volvulus should be reduced or resected. Reduction can be achieved non-operatively by sigmoidoscopy or by hydrostatic decompression with a contrast enema. Volvulus recurrence rate after simple reduction is approximately 50%.
11. **Where is the cancer usually located?**
Ans: In the left colon: Lesions of the right usually do not obstruct, they present with occult bleeding.
12. **Where is the volvulus located?**
Ans: In either the sigmoid colon or the cecum: Right colon or rectal volvulus is a congenital entity caused by failure of the peritoneal attachments you from during the 13th week of gestation. Sigmoid volvulus occurs in the older population when a dietary change causes the sigmoid colon to elongate and become redundant.
13. **What two clinical entities encompasses the diagnosis of inflammatory bowel disease?**
Ans: Crohn's disease and ulcerative colitis, the later being either acute or chronic.
14. **What are some major radiologic differences?**
Ans: Terminal ileal involvement, skip areas, internal fistulas, and thumb printing are all rare or absent in chronic ulcerative colitis but common in Crohn's disease.
15. **Crohn's colitis and chronic ulcerative colitis are often difficult to distinguish clinically. What are some major differences that one note on colonoscopy?**
Ans: The colonic appearance of Crohn's disease is that of focal, predominantly right-sided disease. The mucosa is cobblestone in appearance with transverse ulceratives in affected areas. Biopsies reveal transmural disease with focal granulomas. ON colonoscopy, chronic ulcerative colitis usually appears as a diffuse disease. However, if only a portion of the colon is involved, it is on the left side and almost always the rectum. Pathologic changes involves primarily the mucosa and submucosa.
16. **What are the major indications for surgery in Crohn's disease?**
Ans: It depends on the site of involvement. Enteroenteral fistulae (controversial), abscesses and intestinal obstruction are the most common indications for small intestinal and ileocolic types. Perianal disease and medical failure as well as ileocolic fistulae and abscess formation are the most common indications for surgery in the colonic type.
17. **What is the surgical procedure for the treatment of ulcerative colitis?**
Ans: Total colectomy with formation of a standard ileostomy. Kock pouch, or ileoanal anastomosis (controversial). Ileorectal anstomosis with preservation of rectal has been advocated by some (controversial).
18. **What are the acceptable surgical procedures for the treatment of complications of Crohn's disease?**
Ans: Complication requiring surgeries are usually corrected by removing all areas of bowel involved in the complication. There has been increased experience with stricture plasty as opposed to resection in selected cases of small bowel obstruction (controversial). When

resection is necessary, grossly clear margins are satisfactory. Skip areas are left alone unless they are directly adjacent to resected intestine.

Crohn's disease		*Ulcerative colitis*
Distribution	Small intestine 90% (40–60%)	Small Intestine Backwash Ileitis Rectum Involved
Pathology	Transmural granulomatous inflammation Superficial ulcerations Bowel wall thickened Psuedopolyps uncommon	Inflammation limited to mucosa longitudinal ulcers Transverse Fissures No thickening Pseudopolyps common
Clinical features	Diarrhoea Bowel obstruction Perianal disease	Severe diarrhoea Obstruction rare perianal disease Toxic megacolon
Radiology	Cobble stone mucosa Fistula Fissures	Continuous Involvement Granular mucosa
Endoscopy	Rectal sparing common Cobble stone Mucosa with linear ulcers	Rectum Involved Erythematous mucosa
Treatment	Less responsive High recurrence	Medical treatment 85% Colectomy mucosal proctectomy
Malignancy	<10% after 20 years Small intestine 90% Ileocolitis 40–60%	20–25% after 20 years Small intestine backwash ileitis Rectum involved
Pathology	Transmural granulomatous inflammation Superficial ulcerations Bowel wall thickened Pseudopolyps uncommon	Inflammation limited to mucosa Longitudinal ulcers Transverse fissures No thickening pseudopolyps common
Clinical features	Diarrhoea Bowel obstruction Perianal disease	Severe diarrhoea Obstruction rare perianal disease uncommon Toxic megacolon
Radiology	Cobblestone mucosa Fistulas strictures	Continuous involvement Granular mucosa with ulcers
Endoscopy	Rectal sparing common Cobblestone with mucosa with Clinical ulcers	Rectum involved Erthematous mucosa
Treatment	Less responsive to medical treatment high recurrence rate	Medical treatment 85% colectomy and mucosal proctectomy
Malignancy	<10% after 20 years	20–25% after 20 years

Flow Chart: Lower GI bleeding

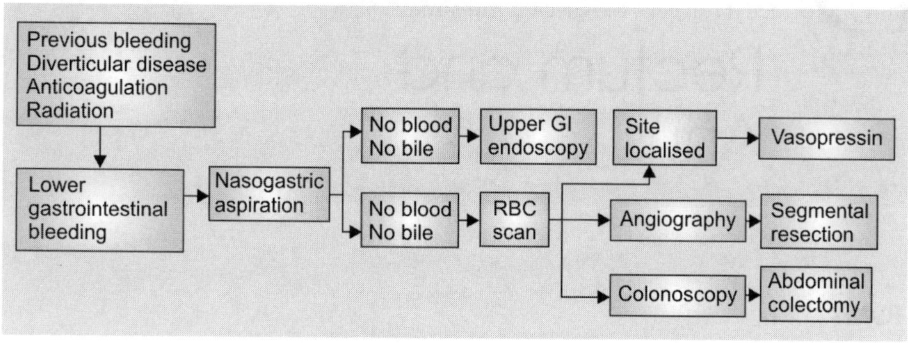

Flow Chart: Ulcerative colon

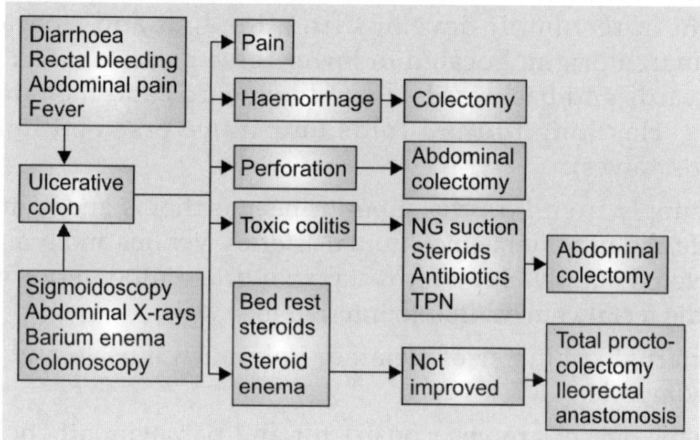

Flow Chart: Carcinoma colon

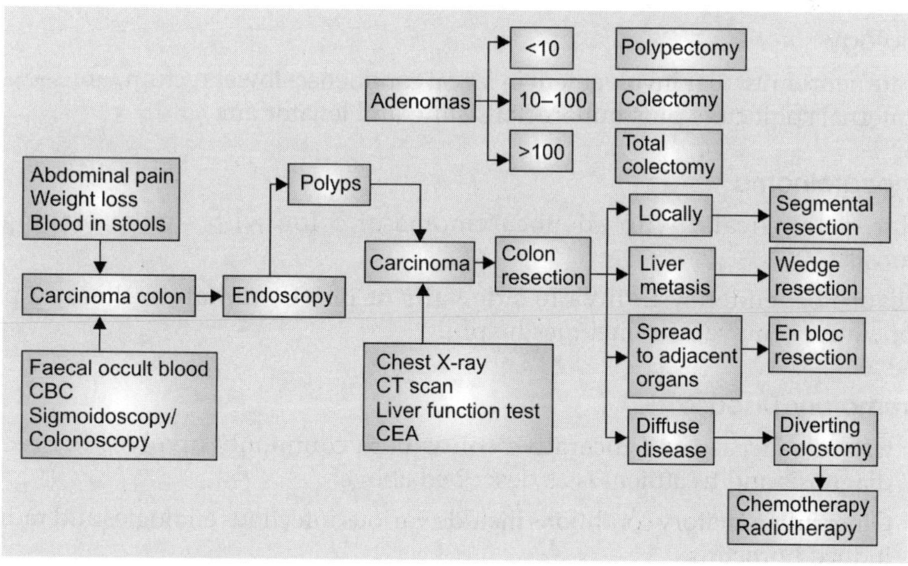

19 Rectum and Anus

ANATOMY

1. Distal part of large gut between sigmoid colon above and anal canal is 5 inches long. Three cardinal features of sacculations, appendices and taenia are absent in rectum. It develops from hindgut and cloaca and both are endodermal in origin. Located in lower three pieces of sacrum and coccyx. It downwards and backwards, then downwards and then downwards and forwards. Has longitudinal folds and transverse and horizontal folds (Houston's valves).
2. Arterial supply from IMA via superior haemorrhoids and from internal iliacs via middle and inferior haemorrhoidal arteries. Venous and lymphatic drainage follow arterial supply. Superior rectal vein drain into inferior mesenteric vein and middle rectal vein drain into internal iliac vein.
3. Outer external sphincter of striated, voluntary muscle and inner smooth, voluntary muscle.
4. Sympathetic nerves are vesoconstrictor and parasympathetic are motor, the rectum and inhibitory to internal sphincter.

Physiology

Intricate neuromuscular involvement in faecal continence–lower rectum/anus–external and internal sphincters plus puborectalis sling and levator ani.

Adenocarcinoma

Similar histologically with adenocarcinoma of colon with similar staging and prognosis.

Because of tendency to invade sidewalls of pelvis, radiation therapy pre or postoperative removal is sometimes helpful.

Inflammatory Disease

1. Crohn's disease and ulcerative colitis both commonly involves the rectum–diagnosis and treatment is as described above.
2. Other inflammatory conditions include various infectious etiologies and radiation induced proctitis.

ANUS

Anatomy/Physiology

1. Terminal portion of large intestine and develops partly from ectoderm (proctadaem) and partly from endoderm (cloacal) extends from anorectal junction to anus and directed downwards backwards. There is external anal sphincter which is made of striated muscle and divided into subcutaneous (surrounds anal canal). Superficial (elliptical surrounds lower parts of internal sphincter and inserted into perineal body. Deep part surround upper part of internal sphincter fused with puborectalis. Internal anal sphincter is involuntary made of 5–8 mm circular muscle and surround upper ¾ of anal canal. Ischiorectal space is on each side of and canal. Perineal space surrounds anal canal below the white line. Submucous space lies above white line between mucous membrane and internal sphincter. Hilton line is situated at level of interval between subcutaneous part of external anal sphincter and lower border of internal anal sphincter and is a felt as a groove in digital examination.
2. Squamous epithelium blends to columnar mucosa at dentate line. Columns of Morgagni between crypts of Lieberkühn secrete mucus.
3. Arterial supply is from superior rectal artery and below pectinate line it is inferior rectal artery. Venous drainage is from internal rectal plexus (haemorrhoidal) lies in submucosa of anal canal. Site of communication between portal and systemic veins. Veins situated in 3, 7, and 11 O'clock position. External rectal venous plexus lies outside the muscular coat and communicates with internal plexus.
4. Above pectinate line anal canal has both sympathetic (inferior hypogastric plexus L1, L2) and parasympathetic (pelvic splanchnic nerves S2, 3, 4) are present. Below pectinate line, it is supplied by somatic (inferior rectal S2, 3, 4).
5. External and internal sphincters control continence and differentiate gas from stool. Internal sphincter is contracted by sympathetic nervous and relaxed by parasympathetic nervous system. External sphincter is supplied by inferior rectal artery.

Congenital Problems

1. Imperforate anus–involves short or long segments of obliterated anus/rectum.
2. Hirchsprung's disease–lack of myomesenteric nerve bodies. (Auerbach and Meissner) leading to poor colonic emptying and an abnormal constricted distal segment of anus/rectum/sigmoid/colon.

Inflammatory Lesions

1. Peri-rectal abscess–obstructed mucous gland at dentate line resulting in an abcess which necessitates to the skin or occasionally will penetrate the sphincteric muscles to invade the ischial space; treated by incision and drainage.
2. Peri-anal fistula often develop after drainage of peri-rectal abcess; Goodsall's rule–cutaneous opening posterior to a horizontal line through the anus usually connect to a posterior midline internal opening, while cutaneous opening anterior to that

line generally run directly straight to a mucosal opening. Treated by opening the tract widely and debriding granulation tissue. (Recurrent lesions could be Crohn's disease).
3. Anal fissures–painful superficial erosions in anterior or posterior midline longitudinal slit in squamous lining of lower anus. Mucosal leaf at external aspect is sentinel pile associated with constipation, especially in children; treated with dilation or sphincterotomy.
4. Perianal warts (condylomata acuminata)–viral etiology, are the most common.
5. Anus soiled due to incontinence poor hygiene, tight pants, thread worm, fistula, dermatoses.
6. Anorectal abcesses are submucous, perianal, intersphincteric, ischiorectal and perirectal. Pain and pyrexia are present.
7. Fistula is abnormal communication between two epithelial lined surfaces. They are superficial, intersphincter, transphincteric and extrasphincteric. When low, they are laid open.

Hemorrhoids (Disrupted Anal Cushions within the Submucosa)

1. Represent dilated veins–external ones are painful, may prolapsed and thrombose or bleed. Internal haemorrhoids are not painful but cause bright red blood on tissue or outside of stool.
2. As there are no surgery fibres above dentate line piles are not painful unless they thrombose. 1° remain in rectum, 2° remain in anus but spontaneously reduce, 3° requires digital reduction, 4° are persistently prolapsed.
3. Most can be treated with local anti-inflammatory agent, local pain, suppressant, diet to reduce strain and constipation (increase fluids, increase bulk, stool softeners, etc.) and sitz baths. Sclerotherapy with phenol, rubber band ligation, cryotherapy, infrared coagulation and haemorrhoidectomy. Thrombosed hemorrhoids, excessive bleeding, severe prolapse all should be excised. Latest treatments is stapler hemorrhoidoplasty.

Neoplasia

1. Epidermoid carcinoma is most common–usually present as, mass lesion, occasionally as fistula that would not heal.
2. Tends to spread into surround soft tissue and femoral/iliac nodes.
3. Reasonably responsive to radiation therapy.
4. Cloacal carcinoma–unusual, squamous, adenocarcinoma, often presents as a submucosal nontender mass and generally poor prognosis.
5. Malignant melanoma may occur in anus–treated like other melanomas.

CA Rectum and Anal Canal

1. Second most commonest carcinoma in males.
2. Complaints of bleeding P/R, diarrhea, alteration in bowel habits, pus, mucosa in anorectum.

3. Detected in 90% cases on digital examination with blood, pus, mucosa in anorectum.
4. Rectal ultrasound to show depth of invasion, lymphadenopathy and abnormal and hepatic metasis, ascites, metastasis lymph nodes, CT scan, MRI scan, EEA and transrectal sound.
5. Types are annular, cauliflower and ulcerative and classification is dukes.
6. Surgical options is anterior resection when tumor is located more than 5 cm from dentate line. Abdominal–perineal resection for tumor located less than 5 cm from the dentate line. Total mesorectal excision (TME) of rectum has become the gold standard for rectal cancer surgery. Convention surgery with chemotherapy (5FU) and radiotherapy does not match with TME results with cure rates as high as 80–87%. Laparoscopic colorectal surgery is also becoming popular specially for non-cancerous lesions. TEM (Transanal endoscopic microsurgery) involves retraction, excision and suturing for smaller tumors done by transanal transacral, trans-sphincteric approach. Rectal cancers are radiosensitive and colonic cancers are chemosensitive.

QUESTIONS AND ANSWERS

1. **What is the dentate line?**

   Ans: The dentate line is an important landmark for surgeons and represents the union of the embryonic ectoderm with the gut endoderm. It is recognizable as the line demarcating the transitional epithelium below and the rectal mucosa above. The columns of Morgagni begin at this line and extend cephalad.

2. **Which types of perirectal abscesses are most disease?**

   Ans: The order of frequency is perineal. Ischiorectal, intersphincteric, and supralevator

Carcinoma rectum TNM	Duke staging
T_q Carcinoma *in situ*	A Growth rectal wall
T_1 Invasion to submucosa	B Growth perirectal fat invading muscularis mucosa
T_2 Invasion to muscularis propria	C_1 Pararectal lymph nodes
T_3 Invasion to subserosa	C_2 Distal lymph nodes
N_1 one to three nodes	D Distant spread
N_2 Three or more nodes	
M_1 Distant spread	

3. **What is treatment for perirectal abscess?**

   Ans: For most patients, particularly those with perineal abscesses, incision and drainage alone is adequate. The primary opening of the anal crypt is rarely identified (35%). The intersphincters abscess is treated by visualizing the bulging area with the anoscope and then performing an internal sphincterotomy over the abscess. Horseshoe abscesses (those surrounding the rectum) are drained through the rectum with counter drains in each ischiorectal space.

4. **What is fistula and predisposing factors?**

   Ans: A fistula is an normal communication between two epithelial lined surfaces. A fistula-in-ano has its external opening into perirectal skin and its internal opening in the anal canal at the dentate line. Predisposing factors high output, Intestinal destruction, short segment, fistula, foreign body radiation, epithelization and neoplasm.

5. **How would the physical locate the internal opening of fistula? What is Goodsall's rule?**

   Ans: Goodsall's rule relates the location of the internal opening to the external opening of fistula-in-ano. If the anus is bisected by a line in the frontal plate, an external opening anterior to the line will connect to an internal opening by a short direct tract. However, if the external opening is located posterior to this imaginary line, the fistula tract follows a curved route to an internal opening in the posterior midline. An exception is an external opening anterior to this imaginary line and greater than 3 cm from the anus, in which case, the tract may cause curve posterior and embedded in the posterior midline.

6. **What is an anal fissure?**

   Ans: An anal fissure is a tear in the anal canal and is frequently associates with sudden pain or bleeding upon defecation. They occur in the posterior midline and may be associated with skin tags or a sentinel pile. Stools softeners are effective is preventing recurrences. Chronic anal fissures may require lateral internal sphincterotomy.

7. **What are hemorrhoids?**

   Ans: The upper anal canal is lined by anal cushions that consist of three thick vascular submucosal bundles that always lie in the left lateral, right posterior lateral, and right anterior lateral position. The function of these cushion is not entirely clear; however, they aid in continence and engorge during defecation to protect the anal canal from abrasion. Haemorrhoids is the pathologic term for a downward displacement of the anal cushions causing dilation of the venules.

8. **What are the most common presenting symptoms of a patient with internal haemorrhoids?**

   Ans: The most common manifestations of internal haemorrhoids is painless, bright red rectal bleeding often associated with a bowel movement. Pateints will notice blood in the stool. On the toilet tissue, or in the toilet. Prolapse of an internal haemorrhoid may produce a mucous discharge causing itching or moisture in the anal region. Buls and Goldberg have outlines a standard classification of haemorrhoidal disease. First degree haemorrhoids bleed, but do not produce through the anal orifice. Second haemorrhoids protrude on straining and then spontaneously reduce. Third degree haemorrhoids occur when digital replacement is necessary after protrusion. Fourth degree haemorrhoids have protruded permanently and cannot be reduced manually. Pain is not a common symptom of internal hemorrhoids unless accompanied with thrombosis or infections.

9. **What is the preferred treatment for external and internal hemorrhoids?**

   Ans: External hemorrhoids are best treated with analgesia and warm soaks. Severe pain requires excision of the entire thrombosed hemorrhoids. Symptoms of bleeding and protrusions of internal hemorrhoids can be controlled by non-operative treatment. Avoidance of constipating food, increasing the fibre of diet, and the use of hydrophilic bulk stool-forming agents can often resolve all symptoms. Rubber-band ligation is a simple outpatient procedure that can be used to treat patients with first and second degree hemorrhoids. Third and fourth degree hemorrhoids, as well as mixed internal-external hemorrhoids, require haemorrhoidectomy.

10. **Where does the bowel distend most on large bowel obstruction, due to carcinoma for instance?**

Ans: In the caecum. Thus caecal tenderness is an indication for urgent surgery to forestall perforation and general peritonitis.

11. **Classify haemorrhoids**

Ans: 1°–piles bleed only
2°–piles bleed and come down with defaecation, but reduce spontaneously
3°–piles permanently prolapsed.

12. **Which types of piles are helped by injection sclerotherapy?**

Ans: Piles which bleed and prolapsed only a little are suitable for injections. Those that prolapsed considerably (especially 3° piles) are suitable.

13. **How should you investigate a patient who receipts painless rectal bleeding without change in bowel habit?**

Ans: The minimum is full history and examination with digital rectal examination, sigmoidoscopy to at least 15 cm and a blood count. If piles are found, treat these, whether all these cases require barium enema is controversial. If no cause can be found, barium enema must be performed.

14. **Compare and contrast the typical features of ulcerative colitis and Crohn's disease**

Ans: **Ulcerative colitis**–presents as bloody diarrhea affects the colon starting at the rectum does not affect the small bowel except rarely the terminal ileum does have a malignancy risk cured by panproctocolectomy with ileostomy. Histology–mucosal disease.

Crohn's disease–presents as episodes of obstruction with slight bloody diarrhea affects small bowel with skip leisons affects large bowel in only 20% tends to keep recurring with complications not pre-malignant, or minimal risk operations only treat the current episodes and are often not curative histology–affects all coats of the bowel.

15. **Compare and contrast the typical presentations of carcinoma of the descending and ascending colon**

Ans: Ascending colon–wide tube with fluid faeces, hence patients presents late. Presents as anaemia or mass.

Descending colon–narrow tube, solid faeces–obstructs early before any mass palpable presents as obstruction or rectal bleeding/change in bowel habit.

16. **What determines whether a patient with rectal carcinoma has an anterior resection retaining the anus, or an abdominal-perineal excision + a permanent colostomy?**

Ans: The site and size of the tumor.

a. You can feel 10 cm inside at P.R. If you cannot touch the cancer, there is room to anastomose below and anterior resection is done. Below 6 cm–most surgeons will do an abdominoperineal resection and permanent colostomy.
b. If the tumor is very large, or fixed , reconstruction after excision may prove impossible.
c. If the tumor is poorly differentiated a more radical excision is usual and this means abdominoperineal operation.

17. **What five symptoms are typical of colonic carcinoma?**

Ans: Change in bowel habit. Passage of blood, slime, mixed up with the stool, abdominal pain, abdominal mass, increasing weakness ± weight loss.

18. What is the usual surgical treatment for acute or chronic ulceratives colitis?

Ans: Acute: Severe acute ulcerative colitis may develop into toxic dilatation of the colon, perforation and death. The key observations are abdominal distention, some tenderness, dilatation of colon on plain X-ray.

19. What are symptoms for colon cancers?

Ans: Right sided colon cancers cause melena and left sides cause haematochezia.

20. What are symptoms of rectal cancers?

Ans: Common symptoms are haematochezia, tenesmus and rectal mass.

21. What is Duke classification for rectal cancers?

Ans:

A	Invasion of submucosa
B	Invasion of muscularis propria
B_2	Invasion of serosa
C	Positive nodal metasis
D	Distant Metasis

22. What is TNM classification for rectal cancers?

Ans:

Stage I	Invades submucosa/muscularis propria
Stage II	Invades muscularis propria
Stage III	Nodes 50%
Stage IV	Distant metasis

23. What are surgical margins for colon cancers and rectal cancers?

Ans: Colon cancers 5 cm proximal, 2 cm distal and rectal cancer 2 cm.

24. What is adjuvant therapy for duke C colon cancers?

Ans: 5-FU and levamisole.

25. What is adjuvant therapy for T_3 and T_4 rectal cancer?

Ans: Radiation, 5-FU.

Flow Chart: Swellings canal

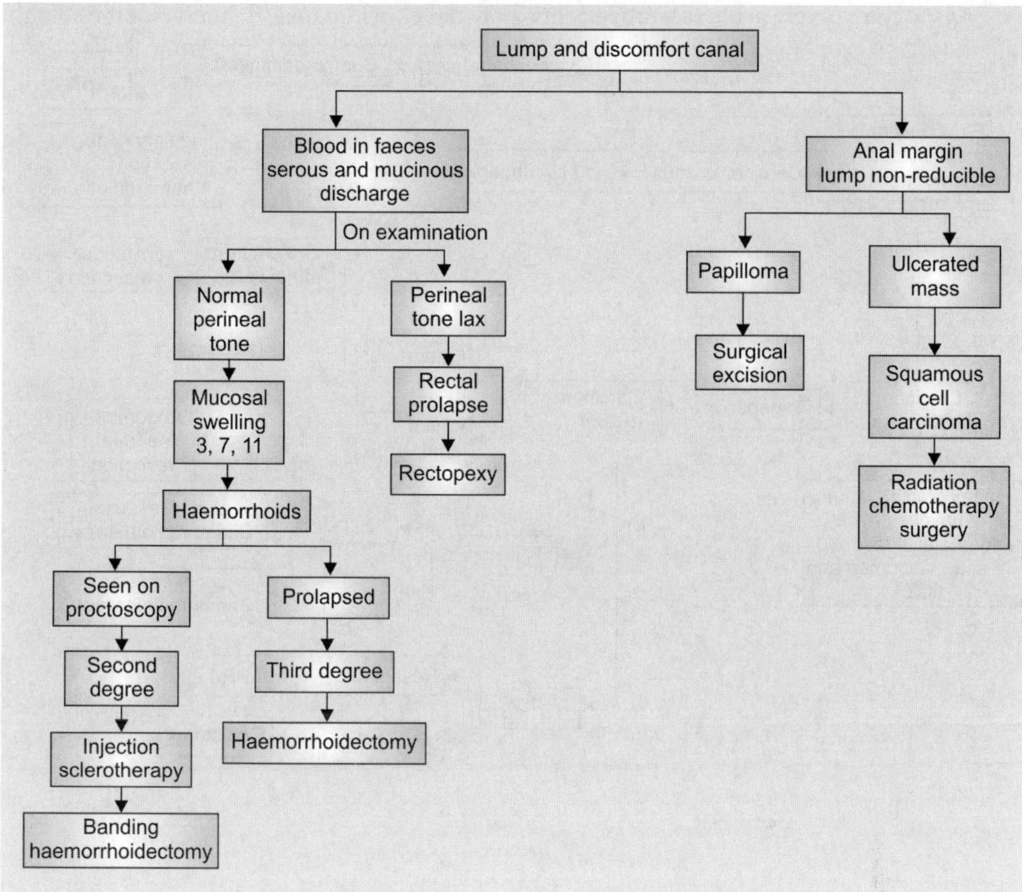

Flow Chart: Swellings anal canal

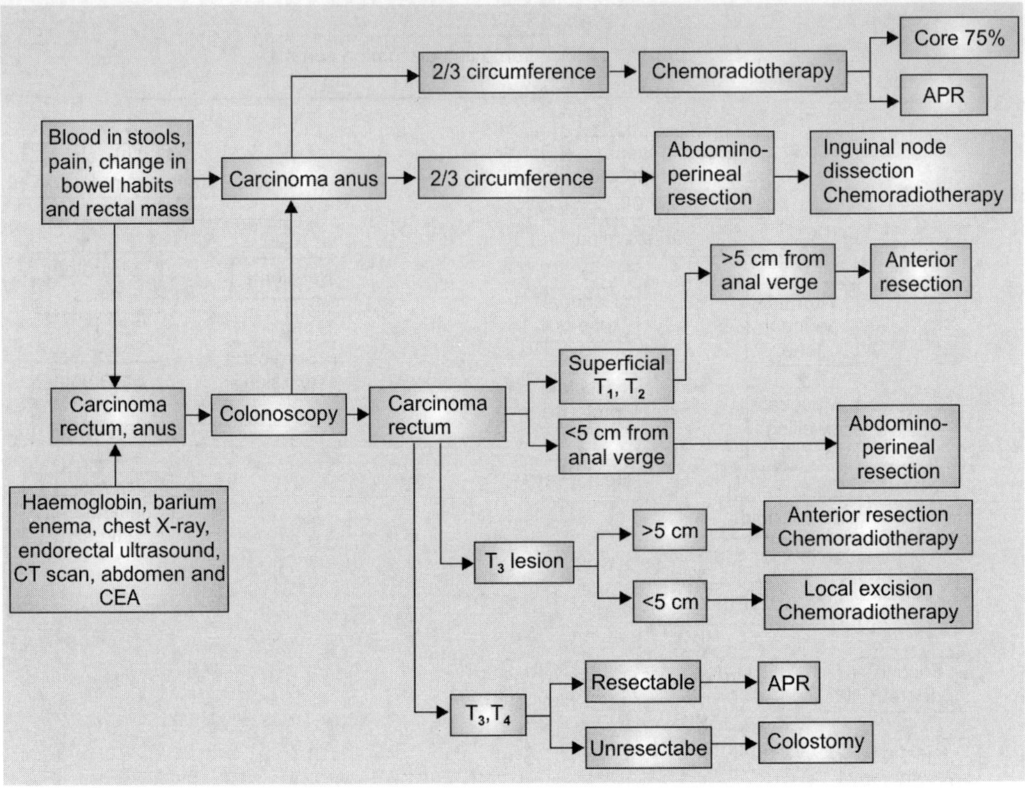

20

Urology

ANATOMY

Kidney

- Extends from upper border of T_{12} vertebra to centre of body of L_3 vertebra.
- Bean shaped 11 cm long 150 gm in adults has two poles, two borders and two surface and before backwards is renal vein, renal artery and renal pelvis.
- Covering of kidney include fibrous capsule, perirenal fat, renal fascia (facia of gerota) consists of anterior layer (fascia of Toldt) and posterior layer (fascia of Zuckerkandl).
- Consists of reddish brown cortex and pale medulla compressed of 1–3 million uriniferous tubules. Secondary part is nephron.
- The renal corpuscles or Malphagian corpuscle.
- Renal tubule
- Collecting duct
- Juxtaglomerular apparatus is formed at vascular pole of glomerulus related to own ascending loop of Henle near distal convoluted tubule consists of macula densa juxtaglomerular cells formed by epitheloid cells and polkisen cells. Granular cells secrete renin which commonest angiotensinogen thus raised blood pressure.
- Arterial supply is by renal artery on each side arising from abdominal which divided into anterior and posterior segmental (end arteries).
- Brodel a vascular line is along lateral border if kidney on its posterior surfaces.
- Venous drainage is by renal vein which drains into inferior vena cava.
- Nerve drainage is by renal pelvis an offshoot of coeliac plexus.
- Normal urine is straw colored (urochrome), 1500 ml/day with specific gravity of (1.1015–1.025).

Ureter

- Narrow thick walled muscular tubes which convey urine from kidney to urinary bladder.
- It is 10 inches long, 3 mm in diameter constricts at pelvic urethral junction, pelvic brim, passage through bladder wall.
- Ureter is supplied by three sets of long arteries upper part from renal, middle from aortic and pelvic from vesical, middle rectal and uterine vessels.
- Ureters is supplied by sympathetic T_{10}–L_2 (ureteric colic) and parasympathetic (S_{2-4}) nerves.

Urinary Bladder

- Muscular reservoir of urine has open connected to umbilicus be median umbilical ligament which represents obliterated embryonic it has base, neck and three surfaces superior and inferolateral.
- Ligaments of bladder include lateral true ligament from bladder to arch of pelvic fascia, puboprostatic from tendinous arch of pelvic fascia to upper part of prostatic sheath medical puboprostatic ligament from to prostatic sheath. In females puboprostatic is known as *pubovesical*.
- Mean capacity of bladder is 200 cm
- Arterial supply is from superior and inferior vesical arteries branches of internal iliac artery. Nerve supply is by vesical plexus derived from nervi erigentes $S_{2,3,4}$ are motor to detrusor and including to sphincter vesicae.
- Sympathetic efferent fibres are (T_{11}–L_2) inhibitory to detrusor and motor. The sphincter vesicae which voluntary hold urine.
- Emptying of bladder is reflex action. Voluntary control is exerted through upper motor nervous and pyramidal tracts. In their lesions voluntary inhibitor and initiation are lost. If spinal reflex is inhibited it leads to retention of urine followed by overflow in continence. When spinal reflux activity returns reflex emptying occurs at intervals (automatic bladder) but it is incomplete residual urine is present.
- If spinal reflex is exaggerated there is precipitancy of micturition. Sensory interruption (tabes dorsalis) leads atonic bladder without any contraction. Lesions of sympathetic motor pathways (lumbar cord lesions) leads to paralysis of sphincter vesicae and dribbling incontinence. Lesions of sympathetic motor (sacral cord cauda equina) causes retention of nerve.
- Ectopia vesicae is developmental anomaly with absence of infraumbilical part anterior abdominal wall, pubis and anterior wall of urinary bladder.

EXTERNAL GENITAL ORGANS

Penis

1. Penis has a root, body and contains superficial fascia of penis of loose areolar tissue and deep fascia or Buck's fascia.
2. Arterial supply is internal pudendal artery is deep artery and artery of bulb.
3. Femoral artery gives superficial external pudendal artery.
4. Sensory nerves are derived from dorsal nerve to penis and ilioinguinal nerve. Parasympathetic ($S_{2,3,4}$) are vasodilator.

Scrotum

1. Cutaneous bag consisting of testis, epididymis and lower part of spermatic cord.
2. Layers include skin, dartos, external spermatic fascia, cremasteric and internal spermatic fascia.

Testis

1. Male reproductive organ 1–1/2" long, weight is 10 to 15 gm.
2. Covering of testis include tunica vaginalis, tunica albuginea and tunica vasculosa.
3. Glandular part of testis consists of semiferous tubules and interstitial cells.
4. Arterial supply is testicular artery. Abdominal vein drains into inferior vena cava on right side and into left renal vein on left side.

Prostate

1. Accessory gland of male reproductive system.
2. Inverted cone weighs 8 gm, separated from anal canal by perineal body.
3. Anterior lobe, posterior lobe, median lobe lies in upper part of and front of ejaculatory ducts. Lateral lobes are on each site of urethra.
4. False capsule has no venous plexus.
5. False capsule–lies outer to true capsule derived from pelvic fascia. Part of it is avascular formed by renovesical fascia of denonvillers.
6. Outer layer zone of branched glands exclusive zone for carcinoma.
7. Inner smaller zone for benign hypertrophy.
8. Nerve supply be prostatic plexus.
9. Blood supply from branches of inferior vesical, middle rectal and internal pudendal arteries.
10. Develop from endodermal buds 1st 3 months of intrauterine.
11. Vertebral plexus of veins is known as **Bateson's plexus.**

Table 20.1: Indication for diagnostic procedure

Procedure	Indication
Cystoscopy	Examination of interior of bladder, examination and evaluation of urethra, including prostatic urethra, for sign of disease process and obstruction; brief urodynamic evaluation to estimate innervations and function of the bladder, facilitation of passage of catheters and stents.
Ureteroscopy	Visualization and extraction of stones in ureter; visualization of questionable areas in ureters or within collecting system of kidney.
Bladder catheterization	Drainage of bladder; measurement of residual urine present immediately following voiding; instillation of contrast material for retrograde cystography and voiding cystourethrography, and radiographic visualization of urethral abnormalities.
Ureteral stenting	Relieve obstruction within the ureter
Prostatic biopsy	Confirmation of diagnosis
Urodynamic studies	Quantitation of functions of detrusor and resistance to overflow of urine to evaluate the physiology of voiding and, more specially and abnormalities of voiding.

Urine Tract Infections

1. Most acute urinary infections are caused by a single bacterial species. Chronic infections are caused by two or more pathogens.

2. Pyelonephritus is ascending infections with obstruction. Treatment is antibiotics after culture.
3. Prostatic caused by sexual activity in women. Treatment is oral antibiotics after culture.
4. Prostatis caused by clamydia trachomatis gram-negative rods. Antibiotics should continue for 4–6 weeks. Prostatodynia is similar with no inflammation.

Haematuria

1. Blood in urine (macroscopic and microscopic) always requires in investigation.
2. Causes are neoplasms of urinary tract, calculi infection, prostatic disease, renal parenchymal disease, trauma and intestinal cystitis.
3. Investigations include urine microscopy, culture cytology, imaging and diagnostic cystoscopy.

Urinary Stone Disease

1. Urinary stones are polycrystalline aggregates of crystals, (90%) mainly calcium, phosphate, oxalate urate and matrix (10%) mainly protein. Stones form in supersaturated urine.
2. Stones types may be calcium (radio-opaque), sterverts (radiolucent), cystene, etc.
3. Clinical presentation include loin to groin colicky pain, haematuria, infection and renal impairment following obstruction:
   a. Investigations include urine and blood examination, pain, haematuria, infection and renal impairment following obstruction:
   b. Treatment involves open or endoscopic removal ureteric stenting lithotripsy or dormia basket extraction. ESWL (extra corporal shock wave lithotripsy and PCNL) are also gaining popularity for smaller multiple renal caculi.

TRAUMA TO THE URINARY TRACT

Mechanisms

1. Deceleration: Especially affects kidney and upper tract
2. Direct injury:
   a. To kidney
   b. To a full bladder predisposing it to rupture
   c. To the perineal urethra
3. Penetrating injury:
   a. From outside the body to any part of the urinary tract
   b. Penetration of the lower urinary tract by a pelvic fractures
4. Indirect injury
5. Iatrogenic injury:
   a. To ureter during pelvic dissection of laparoscopy
   b. To bladder during pelvic surgery or during transurethral procedures

General Management

1. Suspicion of the possibility in sustainable trauma
2. Await micturition
3. Inspect and test urine for blood
4. Appropriate radiology; intravenous urography, cystography and urethrography
5. Bed rest until macroscopic haematuria ceases
6. Blood transfusion and intravenous fluids as necessary
7. Catheter only if essential; if lower tract injury then suprapubic cystostomy
8. Antibiotics

Management at Operation for other Reasons

1. Perinephric hematoma only needs exploration if expanding
2. Urine in the peritoneum: Repair the tear: Drain the bladder/perinephric space.

Radiology

All patient with suspected renal trauma should have an intravenous urogram.

1. Abnormalities demonstrated on urogram:
   a. Mild injury; no abnormality
   b. Moderate injury: Delayed opacification, filling defects due to blood clot in the collecting system spastic calyces, large or blurred kidney outline and extravasation of urine.
   c. Severe injury: Some or all of the collecting system is not visible or there may be total non-opacification.
   d. Extravasation in the lower tract may be demonstrated.
2. Indications for arteriography:
   a. Expanding loin haematoma
   b. Signs of severe injury on intravenous urography
   c. Macroscopic haematuria lasting over 7 days
   d. Later for hypertension or suspected arteriovenous fistula.
3. Findings on arteriogarphy:
   a. Non-filling of all or part of the renal vasculature due to major vessel damage.
   b. Cortical lacerations.
   c. Later arteriogram may show cortical atrophy or areas of ischaemia.

Radioactive hippuran scan may be an alternative method of demonstrating absent blood flow in a kidney.

Cystography is rarely of value since most bladder injuries may be demonstrated clinically. Since it requires catheterisation it may increase damage.

Urethrography is used by some in the early management of urethral trauma but more tend to use it later to demonstrate complex strictures.

Kidney

1. Damage to the kidney rarely needs surgery and may be management conservatively. However, progressive hypovolaemic shock with an expanding

loin haematoma indicates major kidney damage and may need nephrectomy. These patients may not be fit for radiological investigation or need investigation before that can be arranged.

2. Major vessel damage can occasionally be repaired if only the intima is damaged.
3. Segmental injury may be managed by partial nephrectomy.
4. Later surgery may be required for areas of local ischaemia or for secondary hydronephrosis.

Ureter

1. Damage by cutting at operation can usually be repaired primarily.
2. Damage by diathermy may devitalize a segment which needs excising.
3. Damage by penetrating missile may devitalize a segment the size of which can be difficult to determine at primary operation and may need secondary procedure following temporary diversion by nephrostomy.
4. Segment loss at the upper end will require urinary diversion.
5. Segment loss at the lower end may be treated by reimplantation if necessary supplemented by a bladder flap to the psoas.

Bladder

1. Intraperitoneal or extraperitoneal urine leak is not a serious problem for 24 to 48 hours and hence suspected injuries can be safely observed for a period.
2. Intraperitoneal rupture may be repaired and drained with a urethral catheter.
3. Extraperitonal rupture may be repaired and drained suprapubically. The retropubic space is also drained. Spontaneous micturition is awaited or alternatively the urethra may be inspected endoscopically at about two weeks.

Urethra

Many urethral injuries are incomplete and may be rendered by ill-advised instrumentation.

Diagnosis on

1. Mechanism of injury
2. Blood at external urinary meatus
3. Failure to pass urine
4. Palpable bladder

Regimes of treatment

a. Early suprapubic catheter or cystostomy; or await micturition and insert suprapubic catheter if this does not occur. At about two weeks urethroscopy or urethrography. Formal repair over a catheter.
b. Early urethroscopy or urethrography: Partial tear–formal repair over catheter.

RENAL CELL CARCINOMA

80–90% of renal tumours are renal cell carcinomas and arise from proximal tubular epithelium. 5–10% are transitional cell tumours rising from urothelium of renal pelvis. Wilms tumor (nephroblastoma) is most common renal tumor of childhood.

M:F: 2:1 increased incidence in 40 years of age, common in smokers and analgesic abusers.

Presentation with haematuria (60%), loin pain, mass, systemic symptoms like hypertension, fever, anaemia, hypercalcemia called paraneoplastic syndromes.

Spread is local, veins, lymph nodes and lungs (cannon ball secondaries), liver and bone.

Investigations include CT or MRI, IVP, X-ray chest, urine examination, renal arteriography staging is an TNM system:

T_1 : <2.5 cm confined to kidney	N_0 : No regional lymph node
T_2 : >2.5 cm confined to kidney	N_1 : Single <2 cm
T_3 : Extension to renal vein/IVC	N_2 : Single 2–5 cm node or multiple <5 cm
T_4 : Extension beyond Gerota's fascia	N_3 : >5 cm
	M_1: Distant metasis

Treatment

Localised disease: Radical nephrectomy is the standard treatment. Partial nephrectomy to alleviate local symptoms. Chemotherapy and radiotherapy are ineffective.

Transitional Cell Carcinoma of Renal Pelvis and Ureter

1. Tumor is uncommon
2. Presentation is haematuria and hydronephrosis
3. Routine imaging as with other kidney tumors
4. Treatment is nephroureterectomy removing a cuff of bladder around ureteric orifice.
5. Radiotherapy and chemotherapy (M-VAC) may be used in advanced disease.

BLADDER TUMOURS

Aetiology

1. Ingested carcinogens: Particularly relevant to the rubber and dye industries since beta naphthylamine has been shown to cause bladder tumours.
2. Animal experiments have suggested that metabolites of tryptophan may include tumours.
3. Smoking may be related.

Presentation

1. Haematuria
2. Symptoms of cystitis but with a sterile pyuria
3. Cytology on screening in the dye industries.

Assessment

Tumours may arise at multiple primary sites or metastasis throughout the urinary tract, therefore, the whole tract must be examined.

1. Urine culture to diagnose superadded infection and exclude tuberculosis
2. Urine cytology–mainly used for screening
3. Radiography especially intravenous urography which demonstrate
   a. Tumours in the upper tract
   b. Filing defect in the bladder if the tumor is over 3 cm diameter
4. Cystoscopy which enables inspection of:
   a. The size and position of tumor
   b. The nature of the tumor
   c. A preliminary assessment of the degree of invasion and necrosis is an indication of invasion.
5. Biopsy for histologically grading and detection of muscle invasion.
6. Bimanual EUS to assess extent of tumor.

Pathology

1. Benign tumours are very uncommon and to be called such must be composed of entirely normal epithelium.
2. Urothelial tumours: Transitional cell carcinoma is by far the commonest tumor.
3. Metaplastic tumours: Squamous cell carcinoma is uncommon.
4. Glandular tumours: Adenocarcinoma is rare.
5. Mossy' bladder epithelium is almost certainly not precancerous.

Classification of Tumours

There are many classification systems; the simplest are based on histologically grades and on the TNM system (nodes are not accessible for assessment except at open operation)

1. History

Grade	Histology	Usual gross appearance
Low	Well differentiated	Fronded
Intermediate	Moderately differentiated	Fronded and solid
High	Poorly differentiated	Solid

2. TNM system

T_1 : Tumor in mucosa and submucosa	Impalpable at EUA
T_2 : Invasion of superficial muscle	Rubbery thickening
T_3 : Invasion of superficial muscle and to serosa	Hard mass and mobile
T_4 : Invasion of other viscera of spread to pelvic wall	Hard mass and immobile or fixed

Treatment of Transitional Cell Carcinoma

1. Superficial lesions $T_{1,2}$ and some T_3.
   a. Small lesions by transurethral resection or diathermy
   b. Larger lesions by:
      i. Transurethral resection
      ii. Open transvesical excision

        iii. Less commonly partial cystectomy. This is less popular now is used mainly for adenocarcinoma
    c. All patients should be followed up with repeated cystoscopy to treat such recurrences.
2. Large, deep or extensive lesions by combination of surgery, radiotherapy and chemotherapy.
    a. Surgery:
        i. Partial cystectomy
        ii. Total cystectomy with urinary diversion. Very widespread multiple lesions may require extensive surgery up to nephro-uretero-cystoprostato-urethrectomy
        iii. Occasionally complete pelvic clearance is indicated
    b. Chemotherapy:
        i. Local with instillation of surface acting agents, e.g. 'thiotepa'
        ii. Systemic chemotherapy with various agents
    c. Radiotherapy:
        i. Local implantation: Suitable for tumors up to 3 cm diameter and over that size too much necrosis occurs in the centre
        ii. Local infusion of colloidal gold, sodium or bromine salts
        iii. External irradiation by super voltage, cobalt or accelerator units.

Other Techniques

1. Hydrostatic pressure technique of Helmstein. Used for extensive tumors and to control haemorrhage in advanced inoperable tumours.
2. Immunotherapy

METHODS OF URINARY DIVERSION

May be classified as follows

Temporary or permanent
Intubated or non-intubated
Supravesical or vesical

Nephrostomy

1. Lower pole (inferior calyx) nephrostomy by Malecot or dePezzor catheters.
2. Loop nephrostomy with Silastic catheter is especially useful in the following situations:
    a. Small intrarenal pelvis
    b. When nephrostomy drainage is likely to be prolonged as in severe inflammation, stricture or stenosis at ureteropelvic junction
    c. Where it is essential that the nephrostomy tube cannot fall out as in a pyonephrosis of an obstructed solitary kidney.

Loop Cutaneous Ureterostomy

1. Provide temporary diversion usually in neonates or infants with advanced hydro-ureter and hydronephrosis caused by lower urinary tract obstruction (usually posterior urethral valves). These children have severe electrolyte imbalance and uraemia as a result of advanced renal impairment.
2. The loop should be constructed from the dilated and tortuous ureter as close as possible to the ureteropelvic junction to provide effective decompression of obstructed kidneys.
3. Loop ureterostomy should not be closed (by excision of loop and re-anastomosis of ureter over T-tube ureterostomy *in situ*) before optimal anatomical and functional recovery of dilated upper tracts.

Ureterostomy *in situ*

1. Intubation of an unmobilised ureter. Often a simpler alternatives to nephrostomy.
2. May be used as an adjunct to conservative surgical procedures on the upper urinary tract or to relieve the acute anuria of ureteric obstruction cystostomy.

Suprapubic Cystostomy

1. Bladder neck obstruction
2. Urethral trauma
3. Urethral strictures

Uretero-Ureterostomy

1. Indicated for condition involving the distal ureter with a normal contralateral ureter. An alternatives to:
   a. Psoas-hitch and ureteric reimplementation
   b. Bladder flap (Boari) urethroplasty
2. Contraindicated where ureter obstruction is due to malignant disease or irradiation ureteric stricture.

Ileal Conduit

The preferred method of permanent urinary diversion in adults and children, the peristaltic activity of ileum is greater than that of colon ensuring rapid emptying of conduit and preventing of urine stasis, bacterial overgrowth and retrograde urinary infection. Reflux preventing mechanisms (ureteroileal anastomosis) are not attempted, being necessary in reservoirs not conduits. In children with spina bifida there is no agreement has to the best time for urinary diversion.

The stoma should be constructed away from bony prominences, skin creases and scars. Complications include stenosis at ureteroileal anastomosis, stomal stenosis, skin excoriation, conduit calculus formation and, rarely, adenocarcinoma of ileal conduit.

Colon Conduit

1. Because of the thicker wall of the colon, ureters may be anastomosed in an anti-

reflux fashion. Theoretically this should reduce the incidence of postoperative pyelonephritis.

2. Stomal stenosis may occur with the ileal or colonic conduit. Because of the greater diameter of the colon the wider stoma, the incidence of stomal stenosis may be reduced.
3. The colon conduit is probably free from electrolyte disturbance.
4. Following pelvic exenteration (persistent or recurrent neoplasia of cervical endometrium or vagina after irradiation) a colon has the advantaged of avoiding an intestinal anastomosis.

TESTICULAR TUMOR

Testicular tumor is commonest malignancy in younger males, any lump within tunica vaginalis is cancer unless proven otherwise.

Presentation	:	Painless testis lump and infertility
Tests	:	CXR, CT, excision biopsy, alfa fetoprotein, HCG and seminoma (30–40 years) and teratoma (20–30)
Staging	:	1. No incidence of metasis 2. Infradiaphragmatic nodes 3. Supradiaphragmatic nodes 4. Distant metasis
Treatment	:	Orchidectomy by inguinal incision. Seminoma is radiosensitive. Stage-I is treated with orchidectomy with radiotherapy. Response for chemotherapy 3 cycles of bleomycin + etoposide + cisplatin combined with orchidectomy is good for teratoma.

Prostate

1. Benign prostatic hyperplasia.
2. Most common benign tumor in males with increase in stomal and glandular elements of prostate.
3. Testosterone is converted into DHT by 5-alfa-reductase which has increase activity in prostate of men.
4. Obstructive–hesitancy, poor stream, incomplete emptying and terminal dribbling
5. Urgency, frequency, nocturia and urge incontinence.

Investigation

1. PSA, urea, creatinine uroflometry imaging.
2. Treatment–prostectomy–open or TURP, TUNA (Transvascular prostate stents).

PROSTATE CANCERS

- Most common diagnosed malignancy in men
- 60% have locally advanced and 50% have metasis at presentation
- Diagnosis is by DRE, serum PSA and prostatic biopsy.

Staging

T_1 Impalpable on rectal examination
T_2 Tumor confined to prostate
T_3 Extracapsular extension
T_4 Fixed and invades after structures
N_1 Pelvic lymph node <2 cm
N_2 Pelvic lymph node >2 cm
N_3 Pelvic lymph node >5 cm

Localised disease	:	Radical prostatectomy and radiotherapy
Locally advanced	:	Radiotherapy, androgen (orchidectomy, LHRH agonist, flutamide (antiandrogen).

QUESTIONS AND ANSWERS

1. **Why is it important to distinguish between acute pain of urine and chronic painless retention?**
   Ans: Treatment is different. Acute painful retention requires immediate/full decompression by catheter. Painless retention requires more thought. Provided the sensory pathways are intact, the condition indicate a chronic status without urgency. Decomposition should be part of an elective planned therapeutic procedures as rapid decompress in a chronically distended bladder. It precipitates haemorrhage into the urinary tract but also, if there is co-existing uraemia, there may be a profound resultant diuresis.
2. **Define varicocele. Is the define an important diagnosis to make?**
   Ans: Varicosity of the cremasteric and pampiniform venous plexuses. Only in male infertility (treating a varicocele makes the testicle cooler and improves the sperm count) and very rarely a left varicocele may indicate a left hypernephroma (renal cell carcinoma). A large varicocele may also cause a dragging sensation in the scrotum.
3. **What are the symptoms and signs of a ruptured urethra?**
   Ans: Pain, perineal haematoma, blood at the external meatus (remember to retract the foreskin) and urinary retention. Instrumentation can convert a partial into a complete urethral tear.
4. **What may mimic a renal calculus on a plain X-ray?**

Ans:		
	Calcified lymph node	Chip fractured
	Gallstone	Vertebra
	Ingested pill	Calcified adrenal
	Phlebolith	Calcified old
	Ossified tip of T_{12}	Renal tuberculosis
	Calcified splenic	Artefact

5. **Outline your management of a painless unilateral testicular swelling**
   Ans: The majority transilluminate, are cystic, being either hydroceles or epididymal cysts. Those that are solid tests should be explored through a groin incision, and are nearly always tumours. Never be tempted to try aspiration of a solid, enlarged testis. If is malignant, you will encourage local seeding.

6. **You see a boy of eleven in your evening surgery with slight dysuria and a painful, enlarged testicle. What should do?**
Ans: Nil by mouth, and personally contact a senior member of the duty surgical team. All testicular pain in young men and boys should be treated as testicular torsion. For practical purposes, urinary infection does not occur in this age group. If there is a major haematoma it will benefit from decomposition. This boy's testicle should be explored within the hour, looking for torsion.
7. **What is a paraphimosis? Is there any urgency about it? How would you reduce once?**
Ans: When the foreskin in tight, forceful retraction may just coax its edge beyond the glans which pops out in full protraction with the tight neck clasping its corona. This constriction causes swelling of the foreskin and glans, which rapidly becomes vast and oedematous. This is a paraphimosis. Treatment is urgent because it hurts and if not reduced may lead to necrosis. If seen early, sedate the patient, cover the penis with KY jelly and attempt forceful manual reduction. If the fails, administer G.A. and cut the constricting band, and then either convert this to a dorsal slit of the foreskin and circumcision.
8. ***History:*** A 50-year-old female first seen with anemia, thirst, headache and weight loss. She also complained of persistent low grade fever and on close questioning admitted to having mild left flank pain. On physical examination, she appeared pale and a left flank mass could be felt. A faint bruit could be heard over the mass. She admitted to no hematuria or urinary symptoms.

QUESTIONS

1. **The early signs of renal cell carcinoma are**
   (a) Hematuria (b) Pain
   (c) Weakness, anemia and weight loss (d) Mass
2. **In diagnosis a renal mass for a possible malignancy, the following study(s) usually definitive**
   (a) IVP alone (b) Nephrography and ultrasonography
   (c) Arteriography (d) All of these
3. **(T) True of (F) False: An avascular renal lesion shown be arteriography rules out renal cell carcinoma**
4. **Which of the following laboratory findings are occasionally associated with renal cell carcinoma?**
   (a) Elevation of RBC, white cell and platelet count
   (b) Elevation of RBC only
   (c) Elevation of ESR (Erythrocyte sedemantation rate)
   (d) Hypercalcemia
   (e) Plasma testosterone elevation
   (f) Anemia
5. **Preoperative evaluation should indicate the following**
   (a) Inferior venacavography and renal venography
   (b) Liver scan
   (c) Bone scan
   (d) Needle biopsy

6. **(T) True and (F) False: Spontaneous regression of metastatic tumor is not uncommon following nephrectomy for primary carcinoma of the kidney**
7. **The five-year survival rate for carcinoma, the following structures should be resected**
   (a) 5% (b) 20%
   (c) 35% (d) 70%
8. **In nephrectomy performed for renal cell carcinoma, the following structures should be resected**
   (a) Gerota's fascia
   (b) The adrenal gland
   (c) The perinephric fat
   (d) Renal artery before the vein
   (e) Renal vein before the artery
   (f) The ureter and a cuff of bladder at the insertion of the ureter
9. **(T) True or (F) False: Renal cell carcinoma is relatively radioresistant**
10. **Renal cell carcinoma a recurrences in the bladder are common. Therefore, frequent follow-up cytoscopy examination are necessary.**

ANSWERS

1. b
2. c
3. F
4. b, c, d, e, f
5. a
6. F
7. c
8. a, b, c, d
9. T
10. F

11. ***History:* A 27-year-old male presented with a history of noting a mass in the scrotum of two weeks duration. The mass was non-painful and otherwise as asymptomatic. On elevation, he was noted to have a chest lesion of 3 cm in a diameter in the lowest left lobe at the lung. On examination, the scrotal mass did not transilluminate**

QUESTIONS

1. **Since transillumination was not positive, the most likely diagnosis is**
   (a) Tumor of the testis
   (b) Hydrocele
   (c) Epididymitis
   (d) Torsion of the testis
2. **When a tumor of the testis is suspected, the following steps are recommended?**
   (a) Biopsy is always done prior to orchidectomy
   (b) Treatment with antibodies for two weeks to see if resolution is possible from possible epididymitis
   (c) Immediate scrotal orchidectomy should be done without biopsy
   (d) Radiation followed by inguinal orchidectomy
   (e) Inguinal orchectomy with high ligation cord without biopsy

3. The incidence of tumor in the undescended testis is

(a) 1 in 100
(b) 1 in 80
(c) 1 in 200
(d) 1 in 2500

4. Match up the age groups with the cell types of testis tumors

(a) Children	i. Seminoma
(b) Adults in their 40s	ii. Lymphoma
(c) Young adults	iii. Embryonal cell carcinoma
(d) Older adults	iv. Teratocarcinoma
(e) Late adolescents	v. Teratoma

5. Indicate which of the following statement(s) is (are) correct: Seminomas

(a) Occur more commonly on the right
(b) Generally show areas of necrosis
(c) Are especially sensitive to radiation and therefore treated by orchidectomy and radiation?
(d) Are treated by orchidectomy, radiation and retroperitoneal node dissection?
(e) Have an excellent prognosis, 90–95% five-year survival when adequately treated?
(f) Have a relatively poor prognosis, 50–60% despite all forms of treatment?

6. There is an increase in the incidence of testicular tumors in

(a) Brothers and identical twins
(b) Dysgenetic testis
(c) A patient who has already had a testicular tumor
(d) All of these

7. In nonseminoma testicular tumors, the current mode of treatment for metastatic disease involving the lungs is

(a) Supportive only
(b) Radiation
(c) Chemotherapy followed by debulking the retroperitoneal nodes and pulmonary wedge resection of residual chest disease
(d) Chemotherapy and radiation only

8. Which of the following statement are correct assuming currently acceptable therapy has been employed?

(a) The 5-year absolute survival rate of nonseminomous tumours is approximately 75% using surgery, chemotherapy and radiation
(b) The 5-year absolute survival rate of nonseminomous tumors confined below the diaphragm is 85%
(c) The 5-year absolute rate of seminomatous tumours is 95–98%
(d) Most metastases show up in the first 2 years

9. The primary chemotherapeutic agent for nonseminomatous tumours currently being used is

(a) Vincristine
(b) Cytotoxin
(c) Actinomycin D
(d) Methotrexate

ANSWERS

1. (a) 2. (e) 3. (b)

4.

(a) children	:	iii. Embryonal cell carcinoma
	:	iv. Teratocarcinoma
	:	v. Teratoma
(b) Adults in 40s	:	i. Seminoma
(c) Young adults	:	iii. Embryonal cell carcinoma
	:	iv. Teratocarcinoma
(d) Late adolescents	:	iii. Embryonal cell carcinoma
	:	iv. Teratocarcinoma
(e) Older males	:	iii. Embryonal cell carcinoma
	:	iv. Teratocarcinoma
	:	v. Lymphoma

5. (d) 6. (a), (c), (e) 7. (c) 8. (a), (b), (c), (d) 9. (c)

10. *History:* A 5-year male, plastic factory worker, presents with microscopic hematuria found on routine examination. He states that he had no burning on urination or pain. The physical examination was entirely within normal limits. During his evaluation, a small filling defect was noted in the right renal pelvis by excretory urogram

QUESTIONS

1. **The differential diagnosis of hematuria associated with a small renal pelvis filling defect notes on excretory urogram, would include**
   (a) Papillary necrosis
   (b) Fungus disease
   (c) Neoplasm
   (d) Stone
   (e) Blood clot
2. **Indicate which is (are) correct: Squamous cell carcinoma of the renal pelvis**
   (a) Account for 15% of renal pelvic tumours
   (b) May develop in reaction to chronic infection or alone
3. **Which of the following statement is (are) correct?**
   (a) Ureteral tumours present most often as ureteral strictures in males more than 50 years of age
   (b) Ureteral tumours present as haematuria and hydronephrosis in males 50 years of age and older
   (c) Ureteral tumours generally arise in the distal ureter
   (d) All of these
4. **Treatment of renal pelvis and ureteral transitional cell tumours is generally done by**
   (a) Local excision
   (b) Removal of the kidney and ureter with an accompanying cuff of bladder including the ureteral orifice
   (c) Radiation and chemotherapy
5. **(T) True or (F) False: Transitional cell carcinoma of the renal pelvis or ureter is likely to recur in the bladder even several years after the original surgical removal of the primary lesion**

6. **Transitional cell ureteral carcinoma carries a prognosis of**
   (a) 10% 5-year survival
   (b) 50% 5-year survival
   (c) 80% 5-year survival
7. **Diagnosis of ureteral tumor and renal pelvis tumor is made by**
   (a) Urine cytology
   (b) Brush ureteral biopsy
   (c) Excretory urogram
   (d) Retrograde pyelography
   (e) All of these

ANSWERS

1. (a), (b), (c), (d), (e) 2. (a), (b) 3. (d) 4. (b) 5. (T) 6. (a) 7. (e)

8. ***History:* A 64-year-old man presented with a painless, ulcerative lesion of the foreskin of his penis. The lesion measure 1 cm in diameter and involved only the foreskin. On close questioning, the patient admitted to having noticed the lesion for at least six months**

QUESTIONS

1. **The most likely diagnosis is**
   (a) Luetic ulcer
   (b) Transitional cell carcinoma
   (c) Squamous cell carcinoma
2. **The most appropriate treatment(s) for the above case is (are)**
   (a) Excisional biopsy removing the foreskin
   (b) Biopsy followed by a partial penectomy with a 2 cm margin
   (c) Radiation
   (d) Topical 5-FU cream
3. **(T) True or (F) False: Of all forms of cancer, squamous cell carcinoma is the most common histologic type**
4. **If a carcinoma of the penis involves the glands or a corpora, the generally accepted treatment is**
   (a) Radiation
   (b) Partial penectomy, 2 cm margin; bilateral deep groin dissection
   (c) Partial penectomy, 2 cm margin, biopsy of iliac node and if these nodes are negative, superficial groin dissection
   (d) Partial penectomy, 2 cm margin; observation of the inguinal nodes. If nodes enlargement exists and persists, a deep dissection is indicated.
5. **Clinical accuracy in assessing whether inguinal nodes are metastatically involved in approximately**
   (a) 10% accurate (b) 50% accurate
   (c) 75% accurate (d) 90% accurate

(T) True or (F) False

6. **Deep iliac node dissection, in addition to inguinal node dissection, has theoretical advantages. These advantages have been shown to be clinically effective in that there**

is a distinct improvement in statistical survival following combined inguinal and iliac node dissection.

7. **In patients with obvious node metastates in the inguinal region it is probably beneficial to remove the metastases from the groin bilaterally, and provide cover for the femoral vessels to prevent possible hemorrhage from tumor erosion.**
8. **Five-year absolute survival in penile cancer without lymph node involvements is**
   (a) 90% (b) 60%
   (c) 20% (d) 10%
9. **Five-year absolute survival in penile cancer with positive lymph node is**
   (a) 40% (b) 20%
   (c) 2%

ANSWERS

1. (c) 2. (a), (c) 3. T 4. (c) and (d) 5. (b) 6. F 7. T
8. (b) 9. (b)

10. ***History:*** **A 57-year–old male experienced the sudden onset of gross, total, painless hematuria 12 hours prior to visiting the emergency room. A three glass urine was positive in all specimens. This is his first episode of bleeding and when he presents to the emergency room he is still bleeding**

QUESTIONS

1. **The best plan to arrive at a diagnosis is**
   (a) Immediate cystoscopy and subsequent excretory urography
   (b) Immediate excretory urography, cytoscopy after bleeding has stopped;
   (c) Retrograde urethrogram, excretory urogram, cystogram, cystoscopy
   (d) Immediate excretory urogram, immediate cystoscopy
2. **The two most likely cases of haematuria in this patient are**
   (a) Benign prostatic hypertrophy (BPH) and transitional cell carcinoma of the bladder
   (b) Renal stone and urinary tract infections
   (c) Renal cyst and prostatic cancer
   (d) Renal cell carcinoma and renal cyst
3. **The diagnosing and staging of a transitional cell carcinoma of the urinary bladder is best accomplished by**
   (a) Cup biopsy of the tumor
   (b) Bladder washing for cytology
   (c) Cystogram
   (d) Transurethral resection of the bladder flush with the bladder wall; biopsy of the muscle beneath the apparent tumor base.
4. **Match the tumor with the appropriate pre-existing lesion**
   (a) Schistosomiasis i. Squamous cell carcinoma
   (b) Bladder diverticulum ii. Adenocarcinoma
   (c) Extrophy of the bladder iii. Transitional cell carcinoma
   (d) Aniline dye worker

5. A papillary lesion located in the left lateral bladder wall is detected at cystoscopy. It is resected and returned grade II, stage B1. What percentages of lesions in this particular situation will recur?

(a) 5% (b) 10%
(c) 25–50% (d) 100%

6. The patient with the grade-II, stage B1 lesion apparently completely resected, require follow-up. Recommended follow up should be

(a) Cystoscopy once yearly, excretory urography every 18 months
(b) Cystoscopy every three months for eighteen months, every six months for eighteen months and nearly for life with excretory urography at frequent intervals
(c) Urinalysis monthly, cystoscopy when hematuria occurs
(d) Monthly cytology, cystoscopy if cytology is positive

7. The tumor, grade III, stage B_2 recurs (invading deeply into bladder muscle). Which of the following further therapies do you consider appropriate?

(a) Segmental cystectomy (segmental resection of the bladder)
(b) Radical cystectomy and urinary diversion
(c) Simple cystectomy and urinary diversion
(d) Open fulguration of lesion; closure of bladder
(e) External radiation therapy

8. The patient with the grade III, stage B_2 recurrent lesion has agreed to cystectomy. What surgical techniques should be used in an attempt to cure the patient of tumor in addition to removal of the bladder and prostate?

(a) Frozen section studies of the distal ureters prior to implantation into the isolated iliac or colon conduit
(b) Excision of the urachus
(c) Total urethrectomy including the urethral meatus

9. The patient has agreed to the cystectomy. Should adjunctive radiotherapy be employed and if so in what dosage(s)

(a) 4800 rads preoperatively
(b) 2000 rads in five days preoperatively
(c) 4000 rads preoperatively
(d) No preoperatively radiotherapy

10. In the patient who has agreed to the radical cystectomy but has not the total urethrectomy, how do you study the urethra to detect a recurrence?

(a) Retrograde urethrogram
(b) Urethroscopy
(c) Urethral saline washings for cytologic study

11. Twenty-four monthly after the patient had the cystectomy, urethrectomy, etc., and ileal conduit urinary diversion, he develops gross painless hematuria. The most likely diagnosis is

(a) Upper tract urothelial tumor
(b) Renal calculus
(c) Fungal infection

12. Can urine cytology from the ileal conduit prove worthwhile in establishing the diagnosis of recurrences?

(a) Yes (b) No

13. The treatment of choice for a patient who has a renal pelvic transitional cell carcinoma is
- (a) Nephrectomy, urethrectomy, resection of a cuff of the bladder on the ispilateral side including the ipsilateral ureteral orifice
- (b) Local excision
- (c) Radiation therapy
- (d) Nephrectomy and partial ureterectomy

14. If the cause of the hematuria is a ureteral tumor, what is the most likely findings on the excretory urogram?
- (a) Normal ureter
- (b) Hydronephrosis
- (c) Ureteral filling defect
- (d) Nonvisualization of the kidney and ureter on the side of the tumor
- (e) Segmental dilatation of the ureter

15. The treatment of this ureteral transitional cell carcinoma should be
- (a) Nephroureterectomy and cuff resection of bladder
- (b) Partial ureterectomy and anastomosis of the ureter
- (c) Excision of the ureter, replacement with ileum and reimplantation of the ileum in the bladder
- (d) Local radiotherapy

ANSWERS

1. (a), (d)
2. (a)
3. (d)
4. (a) (i)
   (b) (iii)
   (c) (ii)
   (d) (iii)
5. (c)
6. (b)
7. (b)
8. (c)
9. (c)
10. (a)
11. (a)
12. (a)
13. (a)
14. (b)
15. (a)

16. *History:* A 57-year-old asymptomatic male undergoing a routine physical examination is found to nodule 1.5 inches size on the right lateral lobe of the prostate. The examiner feels the nodule is benign

QUESTIONS

1. What would be done?
- (a) Reassess the nodule in one year
- (b) Forget about the nodule
- (c) Biopsy the nodule

2. Among the methods of biopsy available, the poorest method in this situation is

(a) Transrectal biopsy with appropriate rectal cleansing and antibiotics
(b) Transperineal biopsy with antibiotics
(c) Open perineal biopsy
(d) Transurethral biopsy

3. Biopsy is returned adenocarcinoma. The approximate follow-up for this patient is

(a) Excretory urogram
(b) Bone survey
(c) Bone scan
(d) Bone marrow acid phosphatase
(e) Liver scan

4. Assuming all proceeding stages show no evidence of metastatic disease, the next step in this patient should be

(a) Radical perineal prostatectomy
(b) Radical retropubic prostatectomy
(c) Transurethral prostatectomy
(d) External radiation therapy
(e) Pedal lymphangiogram, pelvic lymphadenectomy, then radical surgery or radical radiation therapy

5. The first series of nodes involved in metastatic prostatic cancer are

(a) The common iliac nodes
(b) The periaortic nodes at the renal hilum
(c) The femoral nodes
(d) The obturator and the iliac nodes

ANSWERS

1. (c) 2. (d) 3. (a) 4. (e) 5. (d)

Flow Chart: Testicular mass

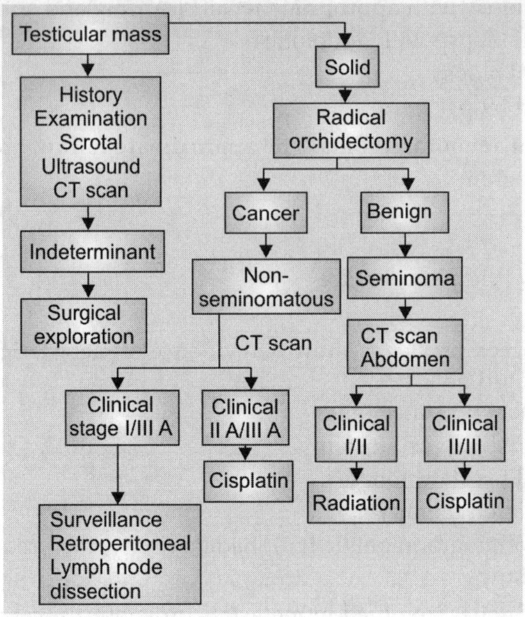

Flow Chart: Nephrolithiasis

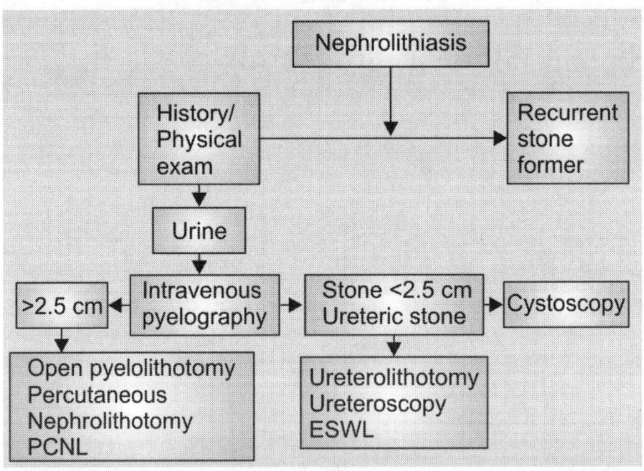

Flow Chart: Haematuria

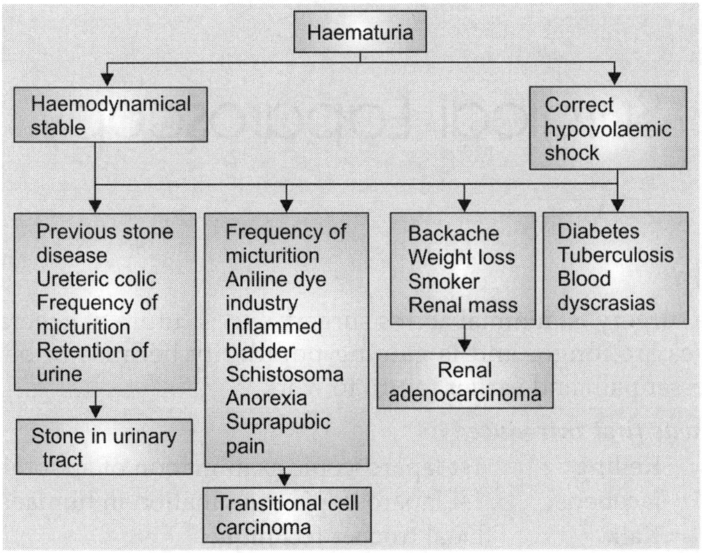

Flow Chart: Scrotal mass

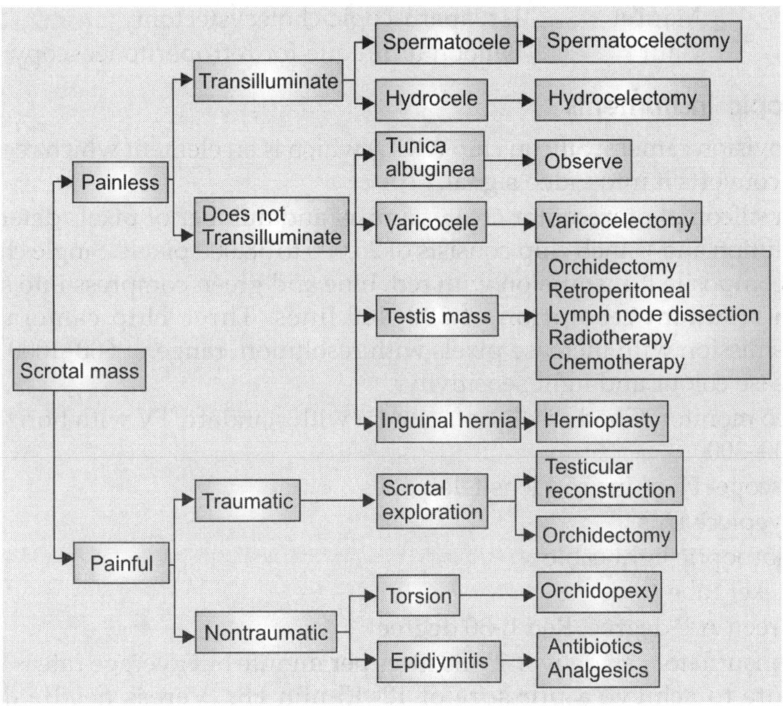

21

Surgical Laparoscopy

LAPAROSCOPY

Term Keyhole surgery is minimal access surgery and is future of general surgery but learning curves are longer and is gaining popularity because of better cosmetic appearance, lesser pain and earlier return to work.

Laparoscopy was first introduced as

1901	Kelling	1st laparoscopic examination of abdominal cavity
1911	Jacobeus	1st laparoscopic examination in humans
1929	Kalk	Dual trocher technique
1938	Veress	Spring loaded obturator
1966	Hopkins	Rod lens optical system
1960–70	Sem	CO_2 insufflator: Laparoscopic instruments
1973	Wittsomar	Laparoscopy for retroperitoneum
1980		TV chip camera
1987	Mauret	1st laparoscopic cholecystectomy
1992	Gaur	Balloon technique for retroperitoneoscopy

Laparoscopic Instruments

- Endovision camera: Silicon chip (CCD) which is an element which receives light and converts it into video signal.
- Each silicon photoreceptor creates a pixel and number of pixels determines the resolution and ½ inch chip consists of 25,000 to 38,000 pixels. Single chip camera has composite transmission with red, blue and green compress into single chip with resultant resolution of 300–400 lines. Three chip camera has RGB transmission with increase pixels with resolution range of 600–1000 lines with increase colour and light sensitivity.
- Video monitor: Good resolution camera with standard TV with horizontal lines of 100–300
- Telescope–Hopkins rod lens telescopes
  a. Eyepiece lens
  b. Fibrooptic light cable
  c. Jacket tube
  Green A-0 degree, Red B-30 degree
- CO_2 insufflator can deliver 15–30 litres per minute but average rate is 9 liters per minute to achieve a pressure of 12–15 mm Hg. Veress needle delivers at

1.5–2 litres per minutes. CO_2 has advantages of being expensive, easily available and suppress combustion, but causes hypercarbia.

- Suction irrigation system–ideal for dissection with simultaneous irrigation and suction 28 cm or 58 cm and 5 mm diameter
- *Energy sources:* Maintenance of laparoscopic instrument either by gas sterilization, chemicals and steam sterilization.

  Laparocopic cholecystectomy is gold standard for treatment of gallstones. indications are:

  a. Symptomatic and asymptomatic cholelithiasis
  b. Acute calculus and acalculus cholecystitis
  c. Gallstone pancreatitis and biliary pain
  d. Gallbladder polyps.

Contraindications

a. Unfit for surgery
b. Coagulopathies
c. Suspected carcinoma of gallbladder.

Laparoscopic appendicectomy has same indications as for open appendicectomy and done with three ports are placed supraumbilical, right and left iliac region. Appendicular artery clipped and endoloop applied at base of appendix.

Laparoscopic groin hernia is becoming the gold standard for treatment of/inguinal/ hernias and specially indicated for recurrent and bilateral hernias. It is done through two routes. Total extraperitoneal repair (TEP) and transabdominal preperitoneal repair (TAPP).

Ventral hernias, splenectomy, fundoplications, nephrectomy, pyelolithotomy, ureterolithotomy, adrenalectomy, sympathectomy, varicocelectomy and illiofemoral bypass are done laparoscopically.

Endosurgery of neck (videoendoscopic neck exploration) has been reported for thyroid and parathyroid pathologies.

Advantages to Laparoscopic Surgery

- Less painful
- Shorter hospital stay
- Faster recovery
- Better
- Better scar

Instruments Used

- Laparoscope
- Light source
- Camera
- Video monitor

- CO_2 insufflator
- Dissecting forceps
- Clip applicators
- Hooks and spatulas
- Needle holders
- Endostaplers
- Veress needle
- Suction irrigation

Physiological Changes due to Pneumoperitoneum due to CO_2 Gas

- CO_2 narcosis
- Sepsis
- Bleeding
- Organ injury
- Subcutaneous emphysema
- Gas emboli
- Postoperative shoulder pain
- Cardiac dysfunction
- Abdominal wall hernia

Laparoscopic cholecystectomy, laparoscopic appendectomy are basic laparoscopic procedures.

Advanced laparoscopic surgeries done are laparoscopic hernia repair

TEP : Extraperitoneal repair

TAPP : Transabdominal repair

Laparoscopic fundoplication, vagotomy, gastrojejunostomy, laparoscopic Nissen's fundoplication, laparoscopic colectomy, hysterectomy, urological surgeries and retroperitoneoscopy.

Laparoscopic Appendectomy

Indications

Acute appendicitis

Camera is at umblical. Two parts are placed, are in lower midline, another at right lumbar region. Appendicular artery is clipped. Endoloop is placed at base of appendix.

- Complications
- Appendicular stump leak
- Pelvic abscess
- Bleeding
- Injury to caecum and ileum
- Diagnostic laparoscopy
- Acute pelvic conditions
- Tubal pregnancy

- Malignancy
- Pain Abdomen
- Retroperitoneoscopy

It is to assess kidneys, ureters, adrenals through retroperitoneal approach, retroperitoneum is expanded by inflating balloon. Different parts are placed.

- Procedures done
- Nephrectomy
- Pyloroplasty
- Adrenalectomy
- Pyelolithotomy
- Retroperitoneal lymph node dissection
- Complications
- Vessel injuries
- Paralytic ileus
- Colon injury

QUESTIONS AND ANSWERS

1. **Who performed the first laparoscopic cholecystectomy?**
   Ans: Eric Muhe Germany performed laparoscopic cholecystectomy in 1985.
2. **Who performed first laparoscopic appendectomy?**
   Ans: Sem performed first laparoscopic appendectomy as prophylaxis.
3. **What is gas used for creating pneumoperitoneum in laparoscopy?**
   Ans: Carbon dioxide.
4. **What are physiological changes due to pneumoperitoneum?**
   Ans: Carbon dioxide causes hypercarbia, acidosis and hypoxia.
5. **What are different telescopes?**
   Ans: 0 degree, 30 degree, 45 degree.
6. **What are different camera systems?**
   Ans:
   1. Single chip camera
   2. Three chip camera
   3. Image 1
7. **What are complications of laparoscopy?**
   Ans: CO_2 narcosis, sepsis, IV compression, bleeding, emphysema, embolism, shoulder pain, cardiac dysfunction, cautery injury to abdominal structure, port hernias and infections.

22 Surgical Radiology and Surgical Complication

1. **What CXR is better?**
   PA view
2. **How much pleural fluid is undetected on CXR?**
   It is said that the diaphragm can overshadow up to 500 cc.
3. **How can CXR confirm that the last hole on a chest tube is in the pleural cavity?**
   The last hole is through the radiopaque line on the chest tube; thus, look for the break in the radiopaque line to be in the rib cage.
4. **How can be loculated pleural effusion be distinguished from a free-flowing pleural effusion?**
   Ipsilateral decubitus CXR; if fluid is not loculated (or contained) it will layer out.
5. **How do you recognize a pneumothorax on CXR?**
   Air without marking is seen outside the white pleural line–best seen in the apices on an upright CXR.
6. **What X-ray should be obtained before feeding via a nasogastric or nasoduodenal tube?**
   Low CXR to ensure the tube is in the GI tract and not in the lung.
7. **What C-spine views are used to rule out bony injury?**
   AP, lateral, open mouth odontoid views.
8. **What plain X-ray are used to look for ligamentous C-spine injury?**
   Lateral flexion and extension C-spine films.
9. **What CXR findings may provide evidence of traumatic aortic injury?**
   Widened mediastinum >8 cm (most common). Apical pleural capping. Loss of aortic knob. Inferior displacement of left main bronchus; NG tube displaced to the right, tracheal deviation and haemothorax.

ABDOMEN

1. **How should an abdominal X-ray (AXR) be read?**
   Check the following:

Patient data:	Name, date, history number up/down, left-right
Orientation technique:	AP or PA, supine or erect decubitus
Air:	Free air under diaphragm, air fluid levels, gas dilatation

Borders: Psoas shadow, preperitoneal fat shadow

Mass: Look for organomegaly, kidney shadow

Stones/calcification: Biliary, faecolith stool, tubes, bones and foreign bodies

2. **How can you tell the difference between a small bowel obstruction (SBO) and an ileus?**

   In SBO there is a transition point (cut-off-sign) between the distended proximal bowel and the distal bowel of normal caliber. The distal bowel may be gasless. The bowel in ileus is diffusely distended.

3. **What is significance of an air-fluid level?**

   Seen in obstruction or ileus on an upright X-ray; intraluminal bowel diameter increases, allowing for generation of fluid and gas.

4. **What are the normal calibers of the small bowel, transverse colon, and caecum?**

   Use the "3, 6, 9 rule." Small bowel <3 cm, transverse colon <6 cm, caecum <9 cm.

5. **What is the rule of 3s for the small bowel?**

   The bowel wall should be less than 3 mm thick. The bowel diameter should be less than 3 cm wide.

6. **How can the small and large bowel be distinguished an AXR?**

   By the intraluminal folds; the small bowel plicae circulates are complete, whereas the plicae semilunaris of the large bowel are only partially around the inner circumference of the lumen.

7. **Where does peritoneal fluid accumulate in the supine position?**

   Morrison's pouch (hepatorenal recess), the space between the anterior surface of the right kidney and the posterior surface of the right lobe of the liver.

8. **What percentage of kidney stones are radiopaque?**

   Approximately 90%

9. **What percentage of gallstones are radiopaque?**

   Approximately 5%

10. **What percentage of patients signs with acute appendicitis have a radiopaque faecolith?**

    Approximately 5%

11. **What are the radiographic signs of appendicitis?**

    Fecolith; sentinel loops; scoliosis away from the right because of pain; mass effect (abscess); loss of psoas shadow; loss of preperitoneal fat strips; and, very rarely, a small amount of free air, if perforator.

12. **What does KUB stand for?**

    Kidneys, ureters, and bladder–commonly used for a plain film AXR.

13. **What is the Parrot's beak or birds beak sign?**

    Evidence of sigmoid volvulus on barium enema; evidence of achalasia on barium swallow.

14. **What are sentinel loops?**
Distention or air-fluid levels (or both) near a site of abdominal inflammation (e.g., seen in RLQ with appendicitis).
15. **What is loss of the psoas shadow?**
Loss of the clear defined borders of the psoas muscle on AXR; loss signifies inflammatory or ascites.
16. **What is loss of the peritoneal fat stripe (AKA preperitoneal fat strips)?**
Loss of lateral peritoneal fat interfaces; implies inflammation.
17. **What is thumbprinting?**
Nonspecific colonic mucosal edema resembling thumb indentations on AXR.
18. **What is pneumatosis intestinals?**
Gas within the intestinal wall (usually means dead gut) that can be seen in patients with congenital variant or chronic steroids.
19. **What is free air?**
Air free within the peritoneal cavity (air or gas should be seen only within the bowel or stomach). Usually results from bowel or stomach perforation.
20. **What is the best position for the detection of free air (free intraperitoneal air)?**
Upright CXR–air below the right diaphragm.
21. **If you cannot get an upright CXR, what is the second best plain X-ray for free air?**
Left lateral decubitus, because it prevents confusion with gastric air bubble; with free air both sides of the bowel wall can be seen; can detect as little as 1 cc of air.
22. **How long after a laparotomy can there be free air on AXR?**
Usually 7 days or less
23. **What is Chilaiditi's syndrome?**
Transverse colon over the liver simulating free air
24. **What should a postoperative abdominal/pelvic CT looking for a peritoneal abscess be performed?**
Postoperative day 7 or later, to give time for the abscess to form.
25. **What is the best test to evaluate the biliary system and gallbladder?**
Ultrasound (US)
26. **What is the normal diameter of the common bile duct with gallbladder present?**
<4 mm until age 40, then add 1 mm per decade (e.g., 7 mm at age 70).
27. **What is the normal common bile duct diameter with acute cholecystitis?**
8 to 10 mm
28. **What U/S findings are associated with acute cholecystitis?**
Gallstones, thickened gallbladder wall (>3 mm), distended gallbladder (>4 cm AP), impacted stone in gallbladder neck and pericholecystic fluid.

SURGICAL COMPLICATIONS

1. **What is Atelectasis?**
Collapse of the alveoli

2. **What is etiology?**
Inadequate alveolar expansion (i.e. poor ventilation of lungs during surgery inability to fully inspire secondary to pain), high levels of inspired oxygen.
3. **What are the signs?**
Fever, decreased breath sounds with rates, tachycardia and increased density on CXR.
4. **What is treatment?**
Postoperative intensity spirometry, deep breathing coughing, early ambulation, postural drainage, suctioning and chest physiotherapy.
5. **What is postoperative respiratory failure?**
Respiratory impairment with increased respiratory rate, shortness of breath, dyspnea.
6. **What is the treatment?**
Supplement O_2, chest PT; suctioning, intubation, and ventilation if necessary.
7. **What is the initial work up?**
ABG, CXR, EKG, monitor and PE
8. **What are indications for intubation and ventilation?**
Cannot protect airway (unconscious), excessive work of breathing, progressive hypoxemia ($PaO_2 < 55$, progressive acidosis (pH < 7.3 and $PCO_2 > 50$) RR > 35
9. **What are the possible causes of postoperative wheezing?**
Diaphragmatic inflammation with possible subphrenic abscess formation, fluid overload and pneumonia.
10. **Why may it be dangerous to give a patient with chronic COPD supplemental oxygen?**
Albuterol nebulizer
11. **Why may it be dangerous to give a patient with chronic COPD supplement oxygen?**
The patient uses relative hypoxia for respiratory drive, and supplement O_2 may remove this drive.

PULMONARY EMBOLISM

1. **What is pulmonary embolism (PE)?**
DVT that embolizes to the pulmonary arterial system.
2. **What is DVT?**
Deep venous thrombosis–a clot forming in the pelvic or lower extremity veins.
3. **Is DVT more common in the right or left iliac vein?**
Left is more common because the aortic bifurcation crosses and possibly compress the left iliac vein.
4. **What are the signs/symptoms of DVT?**
Lower extremity pain, swelling, tenderness, Homan's sign, pulmonary embolus (PE). Up to 50% can be symptomatic.
5. **What is Homan's sign?**
Calf pain with dorsiflexion of the foot seen classically with DVT. But actually found in fewer than one-third of patients with DVT.

6. **What test is used to evaluate for DVT?**
Duplex ultrasonography.
7. **What is Virchow's triad?**
Stasis, endothelial injury, hypercoagulable state (risk factors for thrombosis).
8. **What are the risk factors for DVT and PE?**
Postoperative status, multiple trauma, paralysis, immobility, CHF, obesity, tamoxifen, cancer, advanced age, polycythemia, MI, HIT syndrome, hypercoagulable status (protein C/protein S deficiency).
9. **What are the signs/syndrome?**
Shortness of breath, tachypnea, hypotension, occasionally fever, tender LE, loud pulmonic component of S_2, hemoptysis with pulmonary infarct.
10. **What are the associated lab findings?**
ABG–decreased PO_2 and PCO_2 (from hyperventilation).
11. **Which diagnostic tests are indicated?**
V-Q scan (ventilation-perfusion scan).
12. **What are the associated CXR findings?**
   a. Westermark's sign (wedge-shaped area of decreased pulmonary vasculature resulting in hyperlucency).
   b. Opacity with base at pleural edge from pulmonary infarction.
13. **What are the associated EKG findings?**
More than 50% are abnormal; classic findings is cor pulmonale. EKG most commonly flipped T waves or ST depression.
14. **What is a saddle embolus?**
PE that "straddles" the pulmonary artery and is in both the right and left pulmonary arteries.
15. **What is the treatment if the patient is stable?**
Anticoagulation (heparin followed by long-term [3–6 months] commadin) or Greenfield filter.
16. **What is Greenfield filter?**
Metallic filter placed into IVC via jugular vein to catch emboli prior to lodging in the pulmonary artery.
17. **What is Greenfield filter indicated**?
If anticoagulation or patient has further PE on adequate anticoagulation.
18. **What is the treatment if the patient's condition is unstable**?
Consider thrombolytic therapy; consult thoracic surgeon for possible Trendelenburg operation consider catheter suction embolectomy.
19. **What is the Trendelenburg operation?**
Pulmonary artery embolectomy.
20. **What prophylactic measures can be taken for DVT/PE?**
Heparin (5,000 units every 8–12 hrs; must be started preoperatively). Sequential compression device, compression early ambulation.

23

Chemotherapy, Surgical Signs and Surgical History

Tumor	Effective combination chemotherapies
Acute lymphocytic leukemia in children	Pomp, VP
Acute leukemia in adults	OAP, COAP, Ad-OAP Cooper regimen, CMF,
breast cancer	AC (metastatic)
(Advanced) Hodgkin's disease	MOPP, ABVD
Non-Hodgkin's lymphomas	BACOP, COPP, CVP, CHOP
Multiple myeloma	MP, VBAP, MAP

Abbreviation	*Drugs*	*Doses*	*Frequency*
Hodgkin's disease			
MOPP	M-Mechlorethamine	6 mg/M^2 i.v. days 1+8	
	O-Vincristine (Oncovin)	1.4 mg/M^2 i.v. days 1+8	6 or more
	P-Procarbazine	100 mg/M^2 p.o. days ×14	28-day cycles
	P-Prednisone	40 mg/M^2 days × 14 (for 1st and 4th course only)	
MOP	(same as MOPP except for deletion of prednisone, for previously Mantle field-irradicated patients)		
For MOPP–refractory disease			
CAV	C-Lomustine (CCNU)	100 mg/M^2 p.o. day 1	Repeat cycle
	A-Doxorubicin (Adriamycin)	60 mg/M^2 i.v. day 1	every 6 wk × 9 courses
	V-Vinblastine (Velban)	5 mg/M^2 i.v. day 1	
MVPP	M-Mechlorethamine (HN2) 6 mg/M^2 i.v. days 1–8	14 days cycles	
	V-Velban	6 mg/M^2 i.v. days 1 and 8	with 28-days
	P-Procarbazine	100 mg/M^2 p.o. day 1–14	rest periods,
	P-Prednisone	40 mg/day p.o. days 1–14 of all cycles	usually for 6 or more cycles
ABVD	A-Doxorubicin (Adriamycin)	25mg/M^2 i.v. days 1 and 14	14-day cycles
	B-Bleomycin	10 mg/M^2 i.v. days 1 and 14	with 14-days
	V-Vinblastine	6 mg/M^2 i.v. days 1 and 14	rest periods
	D-Dacarbazine (DTIC)	150 mg/M^2 i.v. days 1–5	
Non-Hodgkin's lymphoma			
COP	C-Cyclophosphamide	800 mg/M^2 i.v. day 1	Cycle
	O-Vincristine (Oncovin)	2 mg i.v. day 1	repeated
	P-Prednisone	60 mg/M^2/days 1–5 orally	at 21 days

(Contd...)

(Contd...)

Abbreviation	*Drugs*	*Doses*	*Frequency*
CVP	C-Cyclophosphamide	400 mg/M²/day × 1–5 p.o.	Repeate
	O-Vincristine	1.4 mg/M² i.v. day 1	at 21 days
	P-Prednisone	100 mg/M²/day × 5	
	(Note : Many CVP and COP regimes exists)		
CHOP	C-Cyclophosphamide	750 mg/M² i.v. day 1	21 days
	H-Doxorubicin (Adriamycin)	50 mg/M² i.v. day 1	cycles
	O-Vincristine (Oncovin)	1.4 mg/M² i.v. day 1 (2 mg max)	
	P-Prednisone	100 mg/M²/day × 5 p.o.	
CHOP-BLEO	CHOP plus Bleomycin	4 unit i.v. days 1 and 8	
CHOP-BCG	CHOP plus BCG (high viability Pasteur)/vial by sacrificing	days 7 and 14	
HOP	CHOP minus cyclophosphamide and doxorubicin increased to	80 mg/M² i.v. day 1	
COPP or MOPP	C-Cyclophosphamide	400 mg/M² i.v. days 1 and 8	28 days
	O-Vincristine (Oncovin)	1.5 mg/M² i.v. days 1 and 8 (2 mg max)	
	P-Procarbazine	100 mg/M² p.o. days 1–14	
	P-Prednisone	40 mg/M² p.o. 3–4 × /day × 10 days	
BACOP	B-Bleomycin	5 mg/M² i.v. days 15 and 21	6 month
	A-Doxorubicin (Adriamycin)	25 mg/M² i.v. days 1 and 8	Cycle
	C-Cyclophosphamide	650 mg/M² i.v. days 1 and 8	
	O-Vincristine (Oncovin)	1.4 mg/M² i.v. days 1 and 8	
	P-Prednisone	60 mg/M² p.o. days 15–29	
COMA	C-Cyclophosphamide	1.5 g/M² i.v.	1–2 wk interval
	O-Vincristine (Oncovin)	1.4 mg/M² p.o. i.v. days 1 and 8	and between cycles
	M-Methotrexate (Leucovorin)	120 mg/M² i.v. days p.o. 25 mg p.o. q 6 hr × 4 (6 hr after methotrexate	8 weekly courses through days 22 to 71
	A-Cytarabine (ARA-C)	300 mg/M² i.v. bolus 16 hr after methotrexate	
Breast Cancer			
Copper's regimen	5-Fluorouracil (5-FU)	12 mg/kg/day × 4 i.v., then 500 i.v.	q wk
	Methotrexate	25–50 mg i.v.	q wk
	Vincristine	0.035 mg/kg i.v.	q wk
	Cyclophosphamide	2.5 mg/kg p.o.	Daily
	Prednisone	0.075 mg/kg p.o.	Daily
CMF	C-Cyclophosphamide	100 mg/M²/day × 14 days p.o.	q 28 days
	M-Methotrexate	40 mg/M²/day i.v. days 1 and 8	
	F-5-Fluorouracil (5-FU)	400 mg/M² i.v. days 1 and 8	
CAF	C-Cyclophosphamide	100 mg/M²/day × 14 days	
	A-Doxorubicin (Adriamycin)	30 mg/M² i.v. days 1 and 8	
	F-5-Fluorouracil (5-FU)	400 mg/M² i.v. days 1 and 8	

(Contd...)

(Contd...)

Abbreviation	*Drugs*	*Doses*	*Frequency*
AC	A-Doxorubicin	30 mg/M^2 i.v. day 1	q 3–4 wk
	C-Cyclophosphamide	150 mg/M^2 p.o. days 3–6	
Malignant Melanoma			
BVD (Note : Many BVD regimens are reported)			
	B-Carmustine (BCNU)	400 mg/day × 3–4	Every 4–6 wk
	V-Vincristine	1.0 mg/day × 3–4	
	D-Dacarbazine (DTIC)	1.0–1.5 mg/wk	
BHD	B-Carmustine (BCNU)	100 or 150 mg/M^2/day × 1 q 6 wk i.v.	Every 3–4 wk
	H-Hydroxyurea	1,480 mg/M^2/day × 5 q 3 wk p.o.	
	D-Dacarbazine (DTIC)	100 or 150 mg/M^2/day i.v. × 5q 3 wk	
	Dacarbazine (DTIC)	850 mg/M^2/day × 1 i.v.	Every 3–4 wk
	Cyclophosphamide	750 mg/M^2/day × 1 i.v.	
	Vincristine	2 mg/M^2 q wk	
DTIC-	Dacarbazine	250 mg/M^2/day × 5 i.v.	
BCG-	BCG vaccine	6 × 10^8	
MeCCNU	MeCCNU	on days 7, 12 and 17	
		100 mg/M^2 p.o. day 1 q 4–6 wk	
Four-drug combination (one of many 4–5 drug regimens reported)			
	Dacarbazine (DTIC)	100 or 150 mg/M^2 days 1–5 q 2 wk	Every 3 wk
	Carmustine (BCNU)	100 or 150 mg/M^2/day × 1q 6 wk	
	Hydroxyurea	1,480 mg/M^2 × 1–5 q 3 wk	
	Vincristine	1.4 mg/M^2 days 1 and 5 q 3 wk	
Lungs cancer			
VAC			
(small livingstone	V-Vincristine	1 mg i.v. day 1	weekly × 12
cell)	A-Doxorubicin (Adriamycin)	50 mg/M^2 i.v. day 1	q 3 wk to
	C-Cyclophosphamide	750 mg/M^2 i.v. day 1	450 mg/M^2 max of Adriamycin
Then			
	Maintenance:		
	C-Cyclophosphamide	1,000 mg/M^2 i.v. day 1	q 4 wk
	M-Methotrexate (Methotrexate)	10 mg/M^2 p.o.	biweekly
	Cyclophosphamide	500 mg/M^2 i.v.	q 3 wk
	Lomustine (CCNU)	50 mg/M^2 p.o.	
(Adrenoepidermoid)			
	Procarbazine	250 mg/day i.v. × 28	
	Flourouracil	10 mg/kg i.v. q.o.d to toxicity	
Bacon			
	B-Bleomycin	30 units i.v. (6 hr after vincristine) q wk × 6	
(squamous cell carcinoma)			

(Contd...)

(Contd...)

Abbreviation	*Drugs*	*Doses*	*Frequency*
	A-Doxorubicin (Adriamycin)	40 mg/M^2 i.v. day 1	q 4 wk
	C-Lomustine (CCNU)	65 mg/M^2 p.o. day 1	q 4–8 wk
	O-Vincristine (Oncovin)	0.75–1.0 i.v. day 2	q wk × 6
	N-Mechlorethamine (nitrogen mustard)	8 mg/M^2 i.v. day 1 (30 min after CCNU)	q 4 wk
Sarcomas			
VAC (standard)	V-Vincristine	2 mg/M^2 (2 mg max) i.v.	q wk × 12
	A-Actinomycin D	0.75 mg/kg/course i.v. × 5 days	q 3 month × 5
	C-Cyclophosphamide	2.5 mg/kg/day p.o. × 2 yr	
VAC (plus)	Same as standard except: Cyclophosphamide	10 mg/kg for 7 days i.v. or p.o.	q 6 wk
CY-VA-DIC			
	CY-Cyclophosphamide	500 mg/M^2 i.v. day 1	
	V-Vincristine	1 mg i.v. (1.5 mg max.) days 1 and 5	
	A-Doxorubicin (Adriamycin)	2 mg/M^2 i.v. day 1 only	
	DIC-Dacarbazine (DTIC)	250 mg/M^2 i.v. days 1–5	
VCR-MTX-CF (osteogenic sarcoma)			
	VCR-Vincristine	2 mg/M^2 (2 mg max.) i.v. × 1	
	MTX-Methotrexate	3,000–7,500 mg/M^2 i.v. as 6 hr	
	CF-Citrovorum factor (calcium leucovorin)	insulin starting 30 min after VCR 15 mg every hr i.v. × 8, then 15 mg p.o. q 3 hr × 8	
Gastrointestinal Tumors			
Advanced colorectal carcinoma			
	Fluororurcil (5-FU)	350 mg/M^2 i.v. × 5	q 5 wk
	MeCCNU	175 mg/M^2 i.v. × 1	q 10 wk
	Vincristine	1.0 mg/M^2 i.v. ×1	q 5 wk
	Flurouracil (5-FU)	400 mg/M^2 i.v. × 1	Weekly
	MeCCNU	175 mg/M^2 i.v. × 1	q 6 wk
Gastric carcinoma			
FAM	F-Fluorouracil (5-FU)	600 mg/M^2/i.v. days 1, 8, 28 and 35	
	A-Doxorubicin (Adriamycin)	30 mg/M^2 i.v. days 1 and 28	every 8 wk
	M-Mitomycin C	10 mg/M^2 i.v. day 1 only	
BCNU plus 5-FU	Carmustine (BCNU)	40 mg/M^2/day /i.v./day × 5	q 6 wk
	Fluorouracil (5-FU)	600 mg/kg/day i.v. × 5	
Pancreatic	Fluorouracil (5-FU)	1 g/M^2/day i.v. days 1 and 8	56-day cycle
	Streptozotocin	600 mg/M^2 i.v. 29, and	every 8 wk
	Mitomycin C	10 mg/M^2 i.v. 36	
Testicular carcinoma			
	Cisplatin	20 mg/M^2/day i.v. × 5	Every 3 wk × 3
	Bleomycin	30 mg i.v.	weekly × 12 wk

(Contd...)

(Contd…)

Abbreviation	*Drugs*	*Doses*	*Frequency*
	Vinblastine	0.2 mg/kg i.v. day 1 and (then 0.3 mg/kg i.v. for maintenance	Every 3 wk Every 4 wk × 2 year
	BCG (Connaught)	1 ampule by scarification after each maintenance Vinblastine	1st, 2nd, and 3rd wk
Uterine Neoplasms			
MOB in Uterin Cervim	M-Mitomycin	20 mg/M² i.v. day 2	q 6 wk
	O-Vincristine (Oncovin)	0.5 mg/M² i.v.	biweekly × 12 wk
	B-Bleomycin	6 mg/M² i.v. (6–12 hr after Vincristine day 1, then	biweekly × 12 wk
AC in Advanced Endometrial	A-Doxorubicin (Adriamycin)	37.5 mg/M² i.v. × 1	Every 3 wk
	C-Cyclophosphamide	500 mg/M² i.v. × 1	
Ovarian Carcinoma			
Hexa-CAF in advanced ovarian carcinoma			
	Hexa-Hexamethylmethenamine	150 mg/M² p.o.	6-months cycles
	C-Cyclophosphamide	days 1 and 14	
	A-Methotrexate	40 mg/M² i.v. days 1 and 8	
	F-Fluorouracil	600 mg/M² i.v. days 1 and 8	
AC-BCG in advanced ovarian carcinoma			
	A-Doxorubicin (Adriamycin)	40 mg/M² i.v. day 1	Repeated at 3–4 week intervals
	C-Cyclophosphamide	200 mg/M² i.v. day 1	
	BCG-Bacillus Calmette-Guerin (Pasteur Institute 6 × 10⁵ c.f.u./vial)	1 vial by scarification on days 8 and 15	
CHAD in advanced ovarian carcinoma			
	C-cyclophosphamide	600 mg/M² i.v. day 1	Repeated q 28 days
	H-Hexamethylmethenamine	150 mg/M² p.o. days 8–21	
	A-Doxorubicin (Adriamycin)	25 mg/M² i.v. day 1	
	D-Cisplatin (DDCP)	50 mg/M² i.v. day 1 with hydration and diuresis	

DRUGS USED FOR CANCER

S. No.	*Name of the drugs packing*	*Amount for one*	*Cycle*
1.	**For head and neck carcinoma**		
	By Cyclophosphamide	500 mg vials	× 1 amp
	By Adriamycin	10 mg vials	× 5 vials
	By Cisplatin	10 mg vials	× vials
2.	**For esophageal carcinoma**		
	By 5-FU	500 mg amp	× 1 amp
	By Adriamycin	10 mg vials	× 5 vials
	By Cisplatin	10 mg vials	× 5 vials
3.	**For Gastric carcinoma**		
	By 5-FU	500 mg amp	× 1 amp
	By Adriamycin	10 mg vials	× 5 vials
	By Mitomycin	10 mg vials	× 5 vials

(Contd…)

(Contd...)

S. No.	Name of the drugs packing	Amount for one	Cycle
4.	**Colorectal carcinoma**		
	By 5-FU	500 mg amp	× amp
	By Adriamycin	10 mg vials	× 5 vials
	By Mitomycin	10 mg vials	× 4 vials
5.	**For breast carcinoma**		
	A. Thermonal H		
	Tab Tamoxifen	10 mg vials	
	B. CMF regime		
	By Cyclophosphamide	500 mg vials	× 1 vial
	By Methotrexate	50 mg vials	× 1 vial
	By 5-FU	500 mg amp	× 1 amp
	C. CAF regime		
	By Cyclophosphamide	500 mg vials	× 1 vial
	By Adriamycin	10 mg vials	× 5 vials
	By 5-FU	500 mg vials	× 1 amp
6.	**For Ca Cervix**		
	By 5-FU	500 mg amp	× 1 amp
	By Adriamycin	10 mg amp	× 5 vials
	By Cisplatin	10 mg vials	× 5 vials
7.	**For endometrial carcinoma**		
	By Adriamycin	10 mg vials	× 5 vials
	By Cyclophosphamide	500 mg vials	× 1 vial
8.	**Testicular cancer**		
	By Cisplatin	10 mg vials	× 3 vials
	By Etoposide	100 mg vials	× 1 vial
	By Bleomycin	15 mg vials	× 2 vials
9.	**For ovarian cancer**		
	By Cisplatin	10 mg vials	× 5 vials
	By Adriamycin	10 mg vials	× 5 vials
	By Cyclophosphamide	500 mg vials	× 1 vial
10.	**For prostatic cancer**		
	Tab Hen Van 100 mg tabs	100 mg tabs	
11.	**For urinary bladder carcinoma**		
	By Cyclophosphamide	500 mg vials	× 1 vial
	By Adriamycin	10 mg vials	× 5 vials
	By Cisplatin	10 mg vials	× 5 vials
12.	**For renal cell carcinoma**		
	By Adriamycin	10 mg vials	× 5 vials
	By Vinblastin	2 mg vials	× 1 vial
	By Bleomycin	15 mg vials	× 1 vial

SURGICAL SIGNS AND SYNDROMES

1. **What are the A, B, C, Ds of melanoma?**
   Signs of Melanoma: A-Asymmetric; B-Border irregularities; C-Color variation; D-Diameter >0.6 cm and dark black color.
2. **What is the Allen's test?**
   Test for patency of ulnar artery prior to placing a radial arterial line. Simply stated, occlude both ulnar and radial arteries with the examiner's fingers with the

patient's hand in a fist; open fist and release ulnar artery occlusion and assess blood flow to hand.

3. **Ballance's sign**
Dullness to percussion in the left flank/LUQ and resonance to percussion in the right flank seen with splenic rupture/hematoma.
4. **Barrett's esophagus**
Columnar metaplasia of the distal esophagus (GERD related).
5. **Battle's sign**
Ecchymosis over the mastoid process in-patients with basilar skull fractures.
6. **Beck's triad**
Seen in patients with cardiac tamponade:
a. JVP
b. Decreased of muffled heart sounds
c. Decreased blood pressure
7. **Bergman's triad**
Seen with fat embolic syndrome:
a. Mental status charges
b. Petechia (often in the axilla/thorax)
c. Dyspnea
8. **Blumer's shelf**
Metastatic disease to the rectouterine (pouch of Douglas) or rectovesical pouch creating a "shelf" that is palpable on rectal examination.
9. **Boas's sign**
Right subcapsular pain resulting from cholelithiasis.
10. **Carcinoid triad**
Seen with carcinoid syndrome:
a. Flushing
b. Diarrhea
c. Right-sided heart failure (FDR)
11. **Charcot's triad**
Seen with cholangitis:
a. Fever (chills)
b. Jaundice
c. Right upper quadrant pain
12. **Chvostek's sign**
Twitching of facial muscles upon tapping the facial nerve in patients with hypocalcemia.
13. **Courvoisier's law**
An enlarged nontender gallbladder seen with obstruction of the common bile duct, most commonly with pancreatic cancer. Note: Not seen with acute cholecystitis because the gallbladder is scarred secondary to chronic cholelithiasis.
14. **Cullen's sign**
Bluish discoloration of the periumbilical area to retroperitoneal hemorrhage tracking around to the anterior abdominal wall through fascial planes (e.g., acute hemorrhagic pancreatitis).

15. **Cushing's triad**
Signs of increased intracranial pressure:
a. Hypertension
b. Bradycardia
c. Irregular respirations
16. **Dance's sign**
Empty right lower quadrant in children with ileocecal intussusception.
17. **Fothergill's sign**
Used to differentiate an intra-abdominal mass from one in the abdominal wall; if mass is felt while there is tension on the musculature, then it is the wall (i.e., sitting halfway upright).
18. **Fox's sign**
Ecchymosis of inguinal ligament seen with retroperitoneal bleeding.
19. **Goodsall's rule**
Anal fistulae course in a straight path anteriorly and take a curved path posteriorly.
20. **Grey Turner's sign**
Ecchymosis of discoloration of the flank in patients with retroperitoneal hemorrhage as a result of dissecting blood from the retroperitoneal.
21. **Hamman's sign/Crunch**
Crunching sound on auscultation of the heart resulting from emphysematous.
22. **Homans's sign**
Calf pain on forced dorsiflextion of the foot in patient with DVT.
23. **Howship-Romberg sign**
Pain along the inner aspect of the thigh; seen with an obturator hernia as the result of nerve compression.
24. **Kehr's sign**
Severe left shoulder pain in patients with splenic rupture (as a result of referred pain from diaphragmatic irritation).
25. **Krukenberg tumor**
Metastatic tumor to the ovary (classically from gastric cancer).
26. **Kelly's sign**
Visible peristalsis of the ureter in response to squeezing or retraction; used to identify the ureter during surgery.
27. **Laplace's law**
Wall tension = pressure × radius (thus, the colon perforates preferentially at the cecum because of the increase radius and resultant increased wall tension).
28. **McBurney's point**
One-third the distance from the anterior iliac spine to the umbilicus on a line connecting the two.
29. **McBurney's sign**
Tenderness at McBurney's point in patients with appendicitis.
30. **Meckel's diverticulum rule of 2s**
Two percent of the population have a Meckel diverticulum, 2% of those are symptomatic; and they occur with in approximately 2 feet of the ileocecal valve.

31. **Mittelschmerz**
    Lower quadrant pain due to ovulation.
32. **Murphy's sign**
    Cessation of inspiration while palpating under the right costal margin the patient cannot continue to inspire deeply because it brings an inflammed gallbladder under pressure (seen in acute cholecystitis).
33. **Obturator sign**
    Pain upon internal rotation of the leg with the hip and knee flexed; seen in patients with appendicitis/pelvic abscess.
34. **Psoas**
    Pain elicited by extending the hip with the knee in full extension, seen with appendicitis and psoas inflammation.
35. **Phaeochromocytoma rule of 10s**
    10% bilateral, 10% malignant; 10% in children, 10% extra-adrenal, 10% have multiple tumors.
36. **Raccoon eyes**
    Bilateral black eyes as a result of basilar skull fracture
37. **Reynold's pentad**
    a. Fever
    b. Jaundice
    c. Right upper quadrant pain
    d. Mental status changes
    e. Shock/sepsis
38. **Rovsing's sign**
    Palpation of the left lower quadrant resulting in pain in the right lower quadrant; seen in appendicitis.
39. **Saint's triad**
    a. Cholelithiasis
    b. Hiatal hernia
    c. Diverticular disease
40. **Silk glove sign**
    Indirect hernia sac in the pediatric patient; the sac feels like a finger of a silk gloves when under the examination finger.
41. **Sister Mary Joseph's sign**
    Metastatic tumor to umbilical lymph node(s).
42. **Virchow's node**
    Metastatic tumor to left supraclavicular node (classically due to gastric cancer).
43. **Virchow's triad**
    Risk factors for thrombosis:
    a. Stasis
    b. Abnormal endothelium
    c. Hypercoagulability
44. **Trousseau's sign**
    Carpal spasm after occlusion of blood to the forearm with a BP cuff in patients with hypocalcemia.

45. **Valentino's sign**
Right lower quadrant pain from a perforated peptic ulcer due to succus/pus draining into the RLQ.
46. **Westermark's sign**
Decreased pulmonary vascular markings on CXR in a patient with pulmonary embolus.
47. **Whipple's triad**
Evidence for insulinoma:
a. Hypoglycemia (<50)
b. CNS and vasomotor symptoms (e.g., syncope, diaphoresis)
c. Relief of symptoms with administration of glucose.

Surgical Syndromes

1. **What is Ogilvie's syndrome?**
Massive nonobstructive colonic dilatation.
2. **What is Gardner's syndrome?**
GI polyps and associated findings of sebaceous cysts, osteomas, and desmoid tumors (SOD); polyps have high malignancy potential (think: a Gardner plants SOD).
3. **What is Peutz-Jaghers syndrome?**
Benign GI polyps and buccal pigmentation (think: Peutz = Pigmentation).
4. **What is Fitz-Hugh-Curtis syndrome?**
Perihepatic gonorrhea infection.
5. **What is SIADH?**
Syndrome of inappropriate antidiuretic hormone (think: Inappropriately increased ADH).
6. **What is toxic shock syndrome?**
Staphylococcus aureus toxin-induced syndrome marked by fever, hypotension, organ failure, and rash (desquamation–Especially palms and soles).
7. **What is toxic shock syndrome?**
Costochondritis of rib cartilage; aseptic (treat with NSAIDs).
8. **What is Plummer Vinson syndrome?**
Syndrome of: (a) Esophageal web; (b) Iron-deficiency anaemia; (c) Dysphagia; (d) Spoon-shaped nails; (e) Atrophic oral and tongue mucosa. Usually occurs in elderly women; 10% develop squamous cell carcinoma.
9. **What is carcinoid syndrome?**
Bronchospasm, flushing, diarrhea, right-sided heart failure (caused by factors released by carcinoid tumor).
10. **What does ARDS stand for?**
Acute respiratory distress syndrome (poor oxygenation caused by leaky capillaries).
11. **What is dumping syndrome**
Delivery of a large amount of hyperosmolar chyme into the small bowel, usually after vagotomy and a gastric drainage procedure (pyloroplasty/gastro-jejunostomy); results in autonomic instability, abdominal pain, and diarrhea.

12. **What is afferent loop syndrome?**
Obstruction of the afferent loop of a Billroth-II gastrojejunostomy.
13. **What is short-gut syndrome?**
Malnutrition resulting from less than 100 cm of viable small bowel.
14. **What is blind loop syndrome?**
Bacterial overgrowth of intestine caused by stasis.
15. **What is Cushing's syndrome?**
Excessive cortisol production.
16. **What is Rendu-Osler-Weber (ROW) syndrome?**
Syndrome of GI tract telangiectasia/AV malformations.
17. **What is Boerhaave's syndrome?**
Esophageal perforation.
18. **What is thoracic outlets syndrome?**
Compression of the structures existing from the thoracic outlet.
19. **What is Munchausen syndrome?**
Self-induced illness
20. **What is superior vena cava (SVC) syndrome?**
Obstruction of the SVC (e.g., tumor, thrombosis)
21. **What is another name for Sipple' syndrome?**
MEN II
22. **What is another name for Werner's syndrome?**
MEN I
23. **What is Trousseau's syndrome?**
Syndrome of deep venous thrombosis (DVT) associated with carcinoma.
24. **What is Mirrizzi's syndrome?**
Extrinsic obstruction of the common hepatic bile duct from a cystic duct gallstone.
25. **What is refeeding syndrome?**
Hypokalemia, hypomagnesemia, and hypophosphatemia after refeeding a starved patient.
26. **What is compartment syndrome?**
Compartment hypertension caused by edema, resulting in muscle necrosis of the lower extremity, seen in the calf; patient may have a distal pulse.
27. **What is HITT syndrome?**
Heparin-induced thrombocytopenic thrombosis (HITT) syndrome; Heparin-induced platelets antibodies cause platelets to thrombose vessels, often resulting in loss of limb or life (also known as "white clot syndrome").
28. **What is Budd-Chiari syndrome?**
Thrombosis of hepatic veins
29. **What is Mendelson's syndrome?**
Chemical pneumonitis after aspiration of gastric contents.
30. **What is Zollinger-Ellison syndrome?**
Gastrinoma and PUD

Surgical History

1. **Identify the following**
   a. First to use antiseptic (carbolic acid)
   Lister (British surgeon)
   b. First to advocate surgical gloves
   Halsted (made by GOODYEAR®)
   c. Father of antiseptic surgery
   Lister (1827–1912)
   d. Father of American neurosurgery?
   Harvey Cushing
   e. Developer of vascular grafts
   DeBakey (his wife hand sewed them!)
   f. Developed electrocautery for surgery with Dr Cushing
   Bovie (1928)
   g. The Mayo Brother's scrub nurse
   Sister Joseph (of St. Mary's hospital)
   h. Developed the cardiopulmonary bypass
   Gibbon
2. **Identify the year the following procedures were first performed and the physician who performed them**

a. Renal transplant	1954;	Murray
b. CABG	1962;	Sabiston
c. CEA	1953;	DeBakey
d. Heart transplant	1967;	Barnard
e. Artificial heart valve	1960;	Starr
f. Liver transplant	1963;	Starzl
g. Total parenteral nutrition (TPN)	1968;	Rhoades
h. Vascular anastomosis	1902;	Carrel
i. Lung transplant	1964;	Hardy
j. Pancreatic transplant	1966;	Najarian
k. Heart-lung transplant	1982;	Reitz
l. First lap chole	1987;	Mouret and Dubois in France
m. First appendectomy	1848;	Hancock
n. First gastrectomy	1881;	Billroth
o. First lap appendectomy	1983;	Semm (Gynaecological Surgery)

3. **Who was the only surgeon to win the Pulitzer Prize?**
   Cushing (for his biography on Osler).
4. **Which surgeons have won the Nobel Prize?**
   Kocher 1909 (Thyroid surgery). Gullstrand 1991 (Ophthalmology). Carrel 1912 (Transplantation/vascular anastomosis). Barany 1914 (Inner ear disease-vestibular disease). Banting 1922 (Insulin). Hess 1949 (Brain physiology). Forssman 1956 (Cardiac catheterization). Huggins 1966 (Oncology). Murray 1990 (Kidney transplant).

24

Surgical Common Diseases and Transplant

SURGICAL MOST COMMON

1. **What are the most common indications for surgery with Crohn's syndrome?**
   Ans: Small bowel obstruction (SBO)
2. **Type is melanoma**
   Ans: Superficial spreading
3. **Type of breast cancer**
   Ans: Infiltrating ductal
4. **Site of breast cancer**
   Ans: Upper outer quadrant
5. **Vessel involved with a bleeding duodenal ulcer**
   Ans: Gastroduodenal artery
6. **Cause of common bile duct obstruction**
   Ans: Choledocholithiasis
7. **Cause of cholangitis**
   Ans: Bile duct obstruction resulting from choledocholithiasis
8. **Cause of pancreatitis**
   Ans: ETOH
9. **Bacteria in stool**
   Ans: Bacteroids fragilis ("B frag")
10. **Cause of SBO in adults in the United States**
    Ans: Adhesions
11. **Cause of SBO in children**
    Ans: Hernias
12. **Cause of emergency abdominal surgery in the United States**
    Ans: Acute appendicitis
13. **Site of carcinoids**
    Ans: Appendix
14. **Abdominal X-ray (AXR) findings with SBO**
    Ans: Air-fluid levels

TRANSPLANT ORGAN

Organ failure is a common action occurrence in some situations can common and in others preserve quality of life and prevent complications.

1. **Autograft**
   Same individually in both donor and recipient
2. **Isograft**
   Donor and recipient are genetically identical (identical twins)
3. **Allograft**
   Donor and recipient are genetically dissimilar, but of the same species
4. **Xenograft**
   Donor and recipient belong to different species
5. **Orthotopic**
   Donor organ is placed in normal anatomic position (liver, heart)
6. **Heterophic**
   Donor organ is placed in a different site than the normal position (kidney, pancreas)
7. **Paratopic**
   Donor organ is placed close to original organ.

BASIC IMMUNOLOGY

Distinct (genetically inherited) cell surface proteins of the human leukocyte antigen (HLA) system.

They are targets (class I antigens) and initiators (class II antigens) of immune response to donor tissue (i.e. distinguishing self from nonself).

All nucleated cells have class I antigens.

Macrophages, monocytes, B cells, activated T cells; endothelial cells have class II antigens.

HLA (human leukocyte antigen) is located in short arm of chromosome and short arm of chromosome 6.

CELLS

T cells is produced in thymus and responsible for cell mediated immunity

1. **What is the function?**
   Ans: Cell-mediated immunity/rejection
2. **What are the types?**
   Ans: (CD4): helper T–help B cell become plasma cells
   Ts (CD8): superior T–regulate immune response
   Tc (CD8): cytotoxic T–kill cell by direct contact

B Cells

3. **What is the function?**
   Ans: Humoral immunity
4. **What is the cell type that produces antibodies?**
   Ans: B cells differentiate into plasma cells

Macrophage: Macrophage is a monocyte in parenchyma tissue. Processes foreign protein and presents it to lymphocytes and known as Antigen-presenting cell (APC)

5. **Briefly describe the events leading to antibody production**
   1. Macrophage engulfs antigen and presents it to Th cells; the macrophage procedure IL-1
   2. The Th cells that produce IL-2, and the Th cell proliferate
   3. The Th cells then activate (via IL-4) B cells that differentiate into plasma cells, which produce antibodies against the antigen presented.

Anastomoses of a heterotrophic kidney transplant

1. Renal artery to iliac artery
2. Renal vein to iliac vein
3. Ureter to bladder

PANCREAS TRANSPLANT

Indications–type-I (juvenile) diabetes associated with severe complications (renal failure, blindness, and neuropathy) or very poor glucose control

For compatibility–ABO, Dr. matching (class II)

Donor requirements

1. 55 years of age or younger
2. Clear chest film
3. PA oxygen tension of 300 on 10% oxygen and 5 cm PEEP
4. No purulent secretions on bronchoscopy.

TRANSPLANT COMPLICATIONS

Note four major complications:

1. Infection
2. Rejection
3. Post-transplant lymph proliferative
4. Complications of steroids

HEART TRANSPLANT

The indications–age birth to 65 years with terminal acquired heart disease–class IV of New York Heart Association classification (inability to do any physical without discomfort =10% chance of surviving 6 months).

The contraindications–older than 65 years of age (variable); active infection; poor pulmonary function and increased pulmonary artery resistance.

Tests for compatibility–ABO, size

Immunosuppression drugs

Cyclosporine, azathioprine (imuran), steroids

Rejection–fever, hypotension or hypertension increased T_4/T_8 ratio.

LUNG TRANSPLANT

Indications

Generally, a disease the substantially limits activities of daily living and is likely to results in death within 12 to 18 months.

Pulmonary Fibrosis

COPD
Eosinophilic granuloma
Primary pulmonary HTN
Eisenmenger's syndrome

Cystic Fibrosis

Indications–current smoking, active infection

1. Which tests comprise the pretransplant assessment of the recipient?

1. Pulmonary–PFTs, V/Q scan
2. Cardiac–echocardiography, angiography
3. Exercise tolerance test.